THROMBOPLASTIN CALIBRATION AND ORAL ANTICOAGULANT
CONTROL

DEVELOPMENTS IN HEMATOLOGY AND IMMUNOLOGY

Other titles in this series:

Thromboplastin Calibration and Oral Anticoagulant Control

edited by

A.M.H.P. van den BESSELAAR, PhD

Reference Laboratory for Anticoagulant Control, Leiden University Hospital, Leiden, The Netherlands

H.R. GRALNICK, MD

Hematology Service, Clinical Center, National Institutes of Health, Bethesda, Maryland, USA

S.M. LEWIS, MD

Department of Hematology, Royal Postgraduate Medical School, Hammersmith Hospital, London, UK

1984 **MARTINUS NIJHOFF PUBLISHERS**
a member of the KLUWER ACADEMIC PUBLISHERS GROUP
BOSTON / THE HAGUE / DORDRECHT / LANCASTER

This publication is based upon a Boerhaave course, organized by the Faculty of Medicine, University of Leiden.

Distributors

---

for the United States and Canada: Kluwer Academic Publishers, 190 Old Derby Street, Hingham, MA 02043, USA
for the UK and Ireland: Kluwer Academic Publishers, MTP Press Limited, Falcon House, Queen Square, Lancaster LA1 1RN, UK
for all other countries: Kluwer Academic Publishers Group, Distribution Center, P.O. Box 322, 3300 AH Dordrecht, The Netherlands

Library of Congress Card Number: 84-1559

ISBN-13: 978-94-010-9005-6   e-ISBN-13: 978-94-009-5676-6
DOI: 10.1007/978-94-009-5676-6

PREFACE

This volume contains all relevant information discussed in a Workshop on thromboplastin calibration held in Leiden, The Netherlands on July 1, 1983. The Workshop was an initiative of the Dutch foundation for a Reference Laboratory for Anticoagulant Control (RELAC) and it was organized by the Boerhaave Committee for postgraduate teaching of the Faculty of Medicine of the University of Leiden. The Workshop was held under the auspices of five organizations i.e. the European Community Bureau of Reference (BCR), the European Committee for Clinical Laboratory Standards (ECCLS), the International Association of Biological Standardization (IABS), the International Committee for Standardization in Haematology (ICSH), and the International Committee on Thrombosis and Haemostasis (ICTH). The aim of the Workshop was to discuss and develop a method for calibration of reagents, i.e. thromboplastins and/or plasmas used for the prothrombin time. During the Workshop three recent thromboplastin calibration studies were discussed, the results of which are presented in chapters 4, 7 and 9. These studies were carried out on the basis of a new calibration model developed by experts working with BCR and WHO. The usefulness of this model and the standardization system based on it is the leading thread running through this volume. Statisticians and clinicians discuss the results from a scientific point of view. Thromboplastin manufacturers, for whom especially the use of the model and the system is intended, discuss the matter also from an economic and legal point of view.

Before the Workshop, one of the commercial manufacturers requested to present data of an additional study in which a newly developed reagent was compared with Manchester Comparative

Reagent. This request was granted (chapter 11) but an editorial comment has been added. Furthermore, Dr. Duxbury, a user of British Comparative Thromboplastin, requested to give his views on thromboplastin nomenclature (chapter 10).

Shortly after the Workshop, in September 1983, the proposed International Reference Thromboplastin human, plain (BCT/253) was accepted by the Expert Committee on Biological Standardization of WHO to replace the original International Reference Preparation, human, combined (code no. 67/40). Thus, the British system of oral anticoagulant control has been intertwined with the WHO system as decribed in chapter 9.

At the conclusion of the Workshop, a draft policy statement for reporting the prothrombin time in oral anticoagulant control was discussed. This policy statement was slightly modified by the ICTH subcommittee for standardization of the prothrombin time at its meeting on July 3, in Stockholm, and was agreed on in principle by both the ICTH and the ICSH. The text given in chapter 14 is the final draft which has been submitted for approval to the members of ICSH and ICTH.

This volume contains a wealth of numerical data and protocols of the calibration studies. This information will be useful to anybody involved in thromboplastin calibration. This includes not only thromboplastin manufacturers, but also anybody concerned with the control of oral anticoagulant treatment.

We thank everybody who contributed to the success of the Workshop, especially Dr. E.A. Loeliger who has been the driving force. We also thank Hellen de Roon, Suzan Leenheer and Emmy Vletter for typing the manuscripts.

November 1983   A.M.H.P. van den Besselaar
                                       H.R. Gralnick
                                       S.M. Lewis

CONTENTS pp.

CONTRIBUTORS

D.J. Baughman
   Ortho Diagnostics, Inc., Raritan, New Jersey, U.S.A.

R.M. Bertina
   Hemostasis and Thrombosis Research Unit, University Hospital, Leiden, The Netherlands

A.M.H.P. van den Besselaar
   Reference Laboratory for Anticoagulant Control, University Hospital, Leiden, The Netherlands

B.McD. Duxbury
   Chase Farm Hospital, Enfield, United Kingdom

B.L. Evatt
   Centers for Disease Control, Host Factors Division, Atlanta, Georgia, U.S.A.

H.R. Gralnick
   Haematology Service, Clinical Center, National Institutes of Health, Bethesda, Maryland, U.S.A.

J. Hermans
   Department of Medical Statistics, University of Leiden, Leiden, The Netherlands

T.B.L. Kirkwood
   National Institute for Medical Research, The Ridgeway, Mill Hill, London, United Kingdom

J.G. Lenahan
   General Diagnostics, Morris Plains, New Jersey, U.S.A.

S.M. Lewis
   Department of Haematology, Royal Postgraduate Medical School,
   Hammersmith Hospital, London, United Kingdom

E.A. Loeliger
   Hemostasis and Thrombosis Research Unit, University Hospital,
   Leiden, The Netherlands

L. Poller
   National (UK) Reference Laboratory for Anticoagulant Reagents
   and Control, Withington Hospital, Manchester, United Kingdom

I. Shirley
   St. Vincent's Hospital, Dublin, Ireland

R. Spaethe
   American Hospital Supply Deutschland GmbH, Department Merz +
   Dade, München, German Federal Republic

J.M. Thomson
   National (UK) Reference Laboratory for Anticoagulant Reagents
   and Control, Withington Hospital, Manchester, United Kingdom

J.A. Tomenson
   National (UK) Reference Laboratory for Anticoagulant Reagents
   and Control, Withington Hospital, Manchester, United Kingdom

D.A. Triplett
   Ball Memorial Hospital, Department of Pathology, Muncie,
   Indiana, U.S.A.

E.A. van der Velde
   Department of Medical Statistics, University of Leiden,
   Leiden, The Netherlands

ACKNOWLEDGEMENTS

The Workshop on thromboplastin calibration was held under the auspices and with contributions of the following agencies:

Community Bureau of Reference of the Commission of European
    Communities
European Committee for Clinical Laboratory Standards
International Association of Biological Standardization
International Committee for Standardization in Haematology
International Committee on Thrombosis and Haemostasis

The generosity of the following manufacturers is gratefully acknowledged for their contributions in support of the Workshop on thromboplastin calibration:

Behringwerke
bioMérieux
Boehringer Mannheim
Ciba-Geigy
Dade Division American Hospital Supply Corporation
Diagnostica Stago
George King Bio-Medical
Hoffmann-La Roche
Immuno Diagnostika
Merz + Dade
Nyegaard
Ortho Diagnostics
Societé d'exploitation de la Technique Biologique
Warner-Lambert Ireland

Chapter 1:   INTRODUCTION

E.A. LOELIGER and A.M.H.P. VAN DEN BESSELAAR

The prothrombin time test is used in oral anticoagulant laboratory control worldwide. However, many different reagents and techniques are applied for this test, and the results are expressed in many different ways. This led to serious misconceptions with respect to the optimal therapeutic range of prothrombin times and with respect to the therapeutic quality control to be applied to maintain high standards of anticoagulation, discrediting the best drug we dispose of in our battle against thrombosis. In our opinion, the medical profession at large and the industry behind it insufficiently recognized that for oral anticoagulants to be effective and safe, the institution of a well-defined level of anticoagulation is mandatory, and that this requires profound knowledge of the drug's pharmacology, the patient's disease state, and the patient's cooperation which should be similar to that operating in haemophiliacs.

As shown schematically in Figure 1, the coagulation defect, initially induced by a so-called loading dose and then continued by a so-called maintenance dose of coumarin, is characterized not solely by the reduction of the levels of factors II, VII, IX, and X in the circulating blood, first at different speeds of disappearance and later (by the 7th day approximately) approaching a level of, for example, about 20 per cent of normal for all four factors, but also by the entrance into the circulation of insufficiently or non-carboxylated and thereby functionally defective precursor molecules (1). These molecules are called PIVKAs, the abbreviation of proteins induced by vitamin K absence and antagonists. Hemker, the father of the PIVKAs, conclusively demonstrated that these proteins strongly interfere with normal

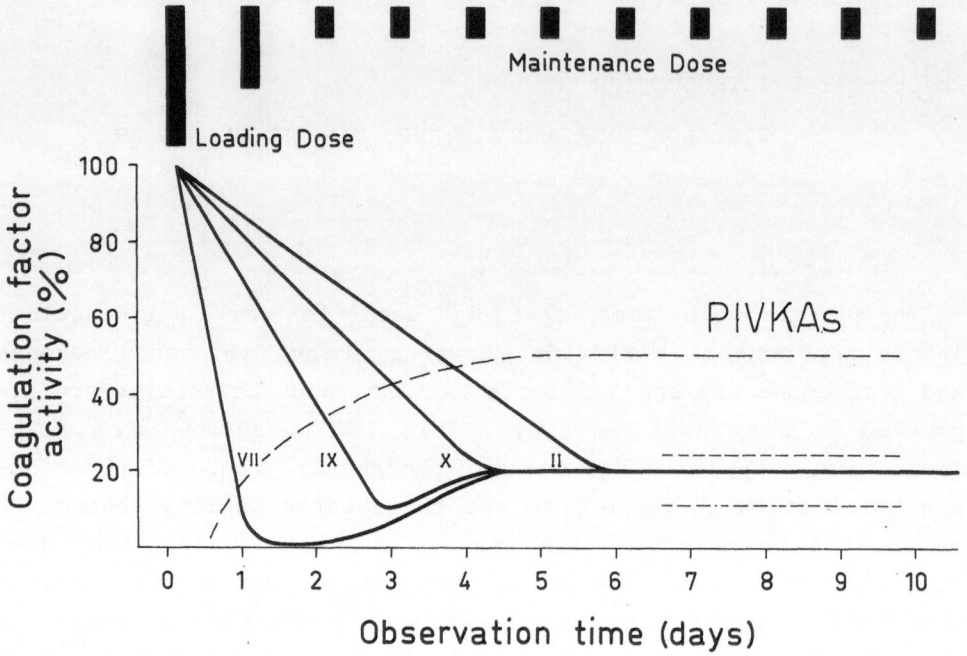

FIGURE 1: Effect of oral anticoagulants on plasma activity of Vitamin K-dependent coagulation factors

coagulation factors in the prothrombin time test using bovine thromboplastin (2). Soon after that, Poller demonstrated the PIVKA sensitivity of human brain thromboplastin (3). And at least some of the rabbit thromboplastins are in all probability PIVKA-sensitive as well (4).

Table 1: Equivalent therapeutic ranges for various thromboplastins expressed in percent prothrombin activity

26 – 37	bioMérieux (rabbit)
16 – 25	Geigy (porcine)
11 – 20	Hepatoquick (rabbit)
5 – 10	Thrombotest (bovine)

Different sensitivity to the PIVKAs of the various thromboplastins and of prothrombin time assay procedures explains why percentages prothrombin activity (Table 1) and by the same token why artificially depleted plasmas cannot be used for international normalization of the prothrombin time. That percentages cannot be used was convincingly demonstrated seven years ago by Duckert (5,6). The studies done by Goguel continue to confirm Duckert's findings (7,8). The fact that neither Duckert's table nor Goguel's data were sufficiently implemented into clinical practice may at least partly be ascribed to the natural reluctance of manufacturers of thromboplastins to refer to recommendations pertaining to competitor thromboplastins in the printed material accompanying their products. Therapeutic failures were its consequence and led to a world-wide disbelief in coumarin therapy for arterial thrombosis, the ambiguous results• of the French Enquête de Prévention Secondaire de l'Infarctus du Myocarde -- the EPSIM study -- being the most recent and perhaps most flagrant example (9,10).

That ratios are equally unsuitable for normalization is shown by the figures presented in Table 2, being, for 12 thromboplastins investigated (Chapter 7), the equivalents to an International Normalized Ratio (abbreviated as INR; see page 5 for definition) or a British Ratio of 3.5. Canadian investigators working at McMaster University in Hamilton are to be credited with having shown irrefutably that the still widely adopted recommendation to prolong the prothrombin time, obtained with particular rabbit thromboplastins, 1.5 to 2.5 times the normal, reflects gross over-anticoagulation at the upper limit of the range (11,12), and that Poller's view (13), since long shared by the Dutch (14,15) and very recently also by American investigators (16), that optimal ranges to be aimed at in venous prophylaxis differ greatly from those in cardiac and arterial prophylaxis, is correct. Prolongation ratios of 1.2-1.5 in terms of many of the rabbit thromboplastins plain are likely to usually be sufficient for venous prophylaxis, while according to Dutch experience values between 1.5 and 2.1 (equivalent to 2.5-5 INR) are

Table 2: Prothrombin time ratios of a number of thromboplastins equivalent to an International Normalized Ratio of 3.5*

thromboplastin (codenumber)	ratio equivalent to INR 3.5
1	1.75
2	1.95
3	1.8
4	1.6
5	1.75
6	2.85
7	1.7
8	1.95
9	3.4
10A	1.75
10B	2.4
11A	3.55
11B	2.55
12	1.85

*for transformation ISIs of the Manufacturers' Calibration Study were used (chapter 7)

needed to be successful in active venous thrombosis and arterial or cardiac prophylaxis (11,15,17,18).

Finally, what holds for prothrombin time ratios holds equally for prothrombin time indices, the latter merely being the inverse of ratios.

This complex situation in oral anticoagulant control with respect to expressing results of the prothrombin time test urged the medical world to find a universally acceptable standardized procedure with which all the modifications could be related. Such a procedure is now available, but the way to find and clarify it was long and its achievement troublesome.

Almost twenty years ago the principle of prothrombin time standardization by means of thromboplastin calibration was developed by Biggs and Denson (19,20) and by Poller (21). This concept implied that one thromboplastin preparation and technique could be used as a reference method with which all other reagents/techniques could be compared. Normalization of the prothrombin time could then be achieved by translation into the reference method scale. In Britain, this approach has been implemented by the introduction of Manchester Comparative Reagent (21), later redesignated the British Comparative Thromboplastin (22,23).

In 1973, the International Committee on Thrombosis and Haemostasis (ICTH) laid down five reference thromboplastins/methods representative for most of the reagents and techniques used worldwide. The National Institute for Biological Standards and Control (NIBSC) in London was the designated custodian of these reference preparations. The preparations were characterized in an international prothrombin time standardization trial in 1974, carried out by an expert panel (chairman: G.I.C. Ingram) appointed by ICTH in collaboration with the International Committee for Standardization in Haematology (chairman: J. Spaander). The results of this trial led to the establishment in 1976 by the World Health Organization (WHO) of one of the ICTH preparations as the International Reference Preparation (IRP) for thromboplastins (ICTH preparation 67/40) against which all thromboplastins had to be calibrated. This preparation, prepared from human brain with the addition of adsorbed plasma as a source of fibrinogen and coagulation factor V, defined the common scale on which prothrombin time test results could be expressed (24). The unit of this scale is the International Normalized Ratio (INR), being the ratio of a patient's prothrombin time to the mean normal prothrombin time when using preparation 67/40.

In 1979, two other ICTH preparations, i.e., bovine thromboplastin (preparation 68/434) and rabbit thromboplastin (preparation 70/178) were established by WHO to be used as reference preparations for bovine and rabbit thromboplastins. The assigned calibration parameters relating them to IRP 67/40 were based on studies by Bangham et al. (25,26).

Several problems were recognized, however (27). First, the stability of IRP 67/40 was questioned by some investigators. Second, IRP 67/40 is not in a form in which human brain thromboplastin is generally used for the control of oral anticoagulant treatment. Third, the WHO preparations were not freely available to manufacturers of commercial thromboplastins.

Responding to these problems and needs, the International Committee for Standardization in Haematology (ICSH) proposed another international calibration study in which the bovine and rabbit WHO preparations, as well as three new reference preparations were to be calibrated against IRP 67/40. The three new preparations included a human brain thromboplastin (batch 099 of British Comparative Thromboplastin), a rabbit brain preparation (RBT/79) and a bovine type preparation (OBT/79). This international study was undertaken in 1979 by the Bureau Communautaire de Référence (BCR) in Brussels (Chapter 4). The experts who cooperated in that study (Table 3) developed a new calibration methodology (described in Chapters 2 and 3) leading to the revision of the WHO requirements by Kirkwood and Lewis (28).

Table 3: Experts cooperating in the thromboplastin calibration study of the Community Bureau of Reference

H. Beeser	Freiburg, D	
B.L. Evatt	Atlanta, USA	
P.T. Flute	London, UK	
H.R. Gralnick	Bethesda, USA	
E.A. Loeliger	Leiden, NL	Laboratory experts
V.G. Nielsen	Herlev, DK	
M. Samama	Paris, F	
L. Tentori }	Rome, I	
M. Orlando		
D.A. Triplett	Muncie, USA	
M. Verstraete }	Louvain, B	
J. Vermylen		
M. Weis Bentzon	Copenhagen, DK	
J. Hermans	Leiden, NL	Statisticians
T.B.L. Kirkwood	London, UK	
E.A. van der Velde	Leiden, NL	
F. Duckert	Basle, CH	
L. Poller }		
J.M. Thomson	Manchester, UK	Advisors
K.J. Stevenson		
F.K. Yee		

In the most recent international study, following the principles of the BCR study, another batch of BCT (BCT/253) was calibrated against IRP 67/40. The study was undertaken in 1983 by the National (U.K.) Reference Laboratory for Anticoagulant Reagents and Control (Chapter 9). This batch of BCT has been accepted by the Expert Committee on Biological Standardization of WHO to replace IRP 67/40.

In practice, national and regional reference laboratories dispose of the WHO reference materials to calibrate national or regional reference thromboplastins, and manufacturers of commercial thromboplastins can calibrate their products against the certified BCR Reference Materials. To test the suitability of the present means of prothrombin time standardization through thromboplastin calibration, twelve European and American manufacturers (Table 4) were invited by the Dutch Reference Laboratory for Anticoagulant Control (RELAC) to cooperate in a pilot study on house standard calibration according to BCR/WHO recommendations, the results of which will be reported on extensively in Chapter 7.

Table 4: Manufacturers cooperating in the house-standard calibration study

Behringwerke, Marburg, D
bioMérieux, Charbonnières-les-Bains, F
Boehringer Diagnostica, Mannheim, D
Ciba-Geigy, Basle, CH
Diagnostica Stago, Asnières, F
Hoffmann-La Roche, Basle, CH
Immuno Diagnostika, Vienna, A
Merz & Dade, Düdingen, CH
Nyegaard, Oslo, N
Ortho Diagnostics, Raritan, USA
Technique Biologique, Paris, F
Warner Lambert, Dublin, EI

The alternative approach to prothrombin time standardization is the use of reference plasmas. However, as long as the biochemical defect induced by coumarin drugs remains ill-defined (see Chapter 13) and long-term stability of lyophilized reference plasmas is not established, this approach remains dependent on reference thromboplastins. However, this alternative developed mainly in connection with proficiency testing surveys in the United States (College of American Pathologists, Centers for Disease Control), in France (Etalonorme) and in Germany (Institut für Standardisierung und Dokumentation im medizinischen Laboratorium), deserves all our attention (see Chapter 12), since, in principle, a survey validated value assigned to a lyophilized plasma sample is an excellent means for any laboratory to calibrate its reagent/method (29,30).

REFERENCES

1. Hemker HC, Veltkamp JJ, Hensen A, Loeliger EA. Nature of prothrombin biosynthesis: preprothrombinaemia in vitamin K-deficiency. Nature 1963; 200: 589-590.
2. Hemker HC, Veltkamp JJ, Loeliger EA. Kinetic aspects of the interaction of blood clotting enzymes. III. Demonstration of an inhibitor of prothrombin conversion in vitamin K deficiency. Thromb Diathes Haemorrh 1968; 19: 346-363.
3. Poller L, Thomson J. The Manchester comparative Reagent. In: H.C. Hemker, E.A. Loeliger and J.J. Veltkamp (eds.), Human Blood Coagulation. Biochemistry, Clinical Investigation and Therapy. Leiden University Press 1969: pp. 290-295.
4. Loeliger EA, Van Halem-Visser LP. Biological properties of the thromboplastins and plasmas included in the ICTH/ICSH collaborative study on prothrombin time standardization. Thromb Haemostas 1979; 42: 1115-1127.
5. Duckert F, Marbet GA. Die Kontrolle der oralen Antikoagulation. Der therapeutische Bereich. Schweiz Rundschau Med 1977; 66: 293-294.
6. Duckert F, Marbet GA. Le controle du traitement aux anticoagulants oraux. La zone thérapeutique. Méd et Hyg 1977; 35: 911.
7. Goguel A. Controle de qualité du temps de Quick. Feuill Biol 1976; 17: 31-43.
8. Goguel A. Confrontation interlaboratoire en hématologie. Etalonorme 81E et 81F (Etalonorme, Association Claude Bernard, 3 Avenue Victoria, Paris IVe. 1981.
9. E.P.S.I.M. Research Group. A controlled comparison of aspirin and oral anticoagulants in prevention of death after myocardial infarction. N Engl J Med 1982; 307: 701-708.
10. Loeliger EA. Oral anticoagulation versus aspirin after myocardial infarction. N Engl J Med 1983; 308: 282.
11. Hull R, Hirsh J, Jay R, et al. Different intensities of oral anticoagulant therapy in the treatment of proximal vein thrombosis. N Engl J Med 1982; 307: 1676-1681.
12. Loeliger EA, Van den Besselaar AMHP, Broekmans AW. Intensity of oral anticoagulation in patients monitored with various thromboplastins. N Engl J Med 1983; 308: 1228-1229.
13. Taberner DA, Poller L, Burslem RW, Jones JB. Oral anticoagulants controlled by the British comparative thromboplastin versus low-dose heparin in prophylaxis of deep vein thrombosis. Br Med J 1978; 1: 272-274.
14. Van der Linde DL. A controlled study of the preventing of thrombo-embolic complications by the use of coumarin derivatives pre-operatively, during the operation and post-

operatively. In: E. Witkins, A.F. de Ruiter, G.L. Stonesifer, J.J. Pflug and J.N. Classen (eds.), Venous diseases, medical and surgical management. Foundation International Cooperation in the Medical Sciences, Montreux 1974: p. 223.

15. Loeliger EA. The optimal therapeutic range in oral anticoagulation. History and proposal. Thromb Haemostas 1979; 42: 1141-1152.

16. Francis CW, Marder VJ, Evarts McC, Yaukoolbodi S. Two-step warfarin therapy. J Am Med Ass 1983; 249: 374-378.

17. Sixty Plus Reinfarction Study Research Group. A double-blind trial to assess long-term oral anticoagulant therapy in elderly patients after myocardial infarction. Lancet 1980; 2: 989-994.

18. Loeliger EA, Lewis SM. Progress in laboratory control of oral anticoagulants. Lancet 1982; II: 318-320.

19. Biggs R. 30th report on the standardisation of the one-stage prothrombin time for the control of anticoagulant therapy. Thromb Diathes Haemorrh 1965; suppl. 17: 303-327.

20. Biggs R, Denson KWE. Standardization of the one-stage prothrombin time for the control of anticoagulant therapy. Br Med J 1967; 1: 84-88.

21. Poller L. A national standard for anticoagulant therapy. The Manchester Comparative Reagent. Lancet 1967; I: 491-493.

22. Thomson JM, Chart IS. The system for Laboratory Control of Oral Anticoagulant Therapy using the British Comparative Thromboplastin. J Med Lab Technol 1970; 27: 207-212.

23. Hills M, Ingram GIC. Monitoring successive batches of British Comparative Thromboplastin. Br J Haematol 1973; 25: 445-451.

24. WHO Expert Committee on Biological Standardization. Twenty-eighth Report. WHO Technical Report Series 610. WHO, Geneva 1977: pp. 14-15 and 45-51.

25. Bangham DR, Biggs R, Brozovic M, Denson KWE. Draft report of a collaborative study of two thromboplastins (including the use of common abnormal plasma). Thromb Diathes Haemorrh 1970; suppl. 40: 341-351.

26. Bangham DR, Biggs R, Brozovic M, Denson KWE. Calibration of five different thromboplastins, using fresh and freeze-dried plasma. Thromb Diathes Haemorrh 1973; 29: 228-229.

27. Ingram GIC. The stability of WHO Reference Thromboplastin NIBS&C 67/40. Thromb Haemostas 1979; 42: 1135-1140.

28. WHO Expert Committee on Biological Standardization. 33rd Report. WHO Technical Report Series 687. World Health Organization, Geneva 1983: pp. 81-105.

29. Koepke JA, Gilmer PR, Triplett DA, O'Sullivan MB. The prediction of prothrombin time system performance using secondary standards. Amer J Clin Pathol 1977; 68: 191-194.

30. Koepke JA. Use of survey validated plasmas as a means of prothrombin time standardization. In: D.A. Triplett (ed.), Standardization of Coagulation Assays: An Overview. College of American Pathologists, Skokie Illinois 1982: pp. 105-110.

Chapter 2:   GENERAL ASPECTS OF THROMBOPLASTIN CALIBRATION

T.B.L. KIRKWOOD

INTRODUCTION

The concept of calibrating preparations of thromboplastins in terms of a single primary reference preparation was suggested sixteen years ago by Biggs and Denson (2). The aim was to permit effective standardisation of prothrombin time (PT) determinations made to monitor the degree of anticoagulation in patients treated with oral anticoagulants. Biggs and Denson (2) asserted: "A single scale properly applied at different centres would ensure safety and uniform dosage for a patient moving from one place to another and would greatly improve the standard of clinical trials carried out at more than one centre".

The scheme which Biggs and Denson (2) proposed was to standardise PT ratios (that is, the patient's PT divided by the average PT for normal plasma) on the grounds that by using the PT ratio instead of the PT alone part of the technical variation in the test is eliminated, the ratio being unaffected if both the patient's and the normal PT vary in the same proportion. Their method was based on the observation that if the PT ratios for a set of patients' plasmas measured with two thromboplastins are plotted against one another (Fig. 1), an approximately straight line relationship is observed. The relationship would be expected to pass through the point (1,1) (equivalent to zero prolongation of the PT with both thromboplastins), so the line could be described by the equation

$$y - 1 = b(x - 1) \qquad\qquad \text{(Equation 1)}$$

where x and y refer to PT ratio values of the horizontal and vertical lines respectively, and b is the slope. Equation 1 has been used as the basis of an international scheme for the cali-

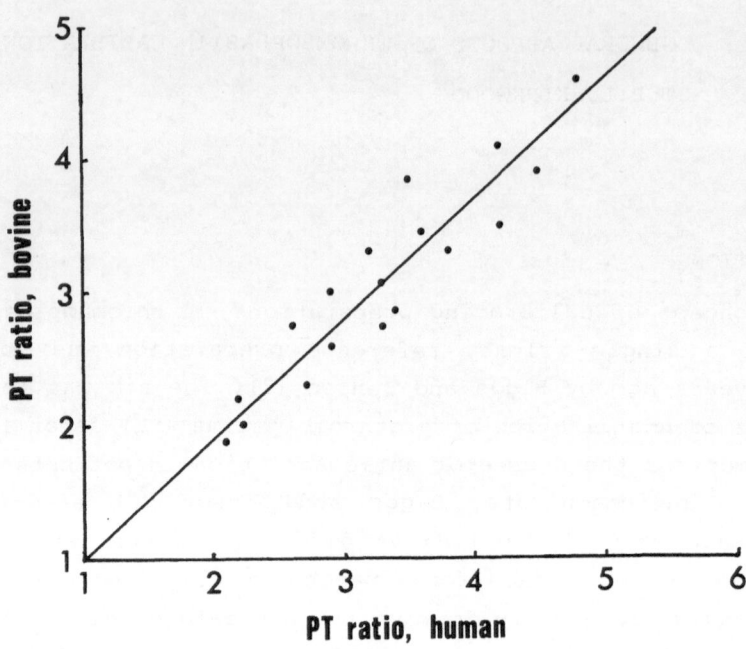

FIGURE 1. PT ratio plot of data for 18 patients obtained using a bovine thromboplastin (vertical axis) and a human thromboplastin (horizontal axis). The Biggs-Denson calibration procedure was based on fitting a straight line passing through the (1,1) origin.

bration of reference thromboplastins which was adopted by the Expert Committee on Biological Standardisation of the World Health Organisation in 1977 (11,12).

In recent years, however, certain difficulties with the calibration model based on equation 1 have come to light (8). Firstly, it appears that there are important instances where the assumption of a straight line relationship through the point (1,1) is not valid (1,3,7). Secondly, there are theoretical difficulties in defining satisfactory statistical procedures, comparable to those which apply in other areas of biological standardisation, where the calibration line must be fitted to ratios for which the numerator (patient's PT) and denominator (normal PT) are both subject to error, but in different ways. While the error in the patient's PT contributes straightforwardly to the scatter in Figure 1, the error in the normal PTs moves the true origin of the calibration relationship away from the point (1,1) by an unknown amount. For these reasons, the calibration model on which the WHO scheme is based has recently been modified (13), and the remainder of this paper is concerned with describing the revised scheme (8).

THE NEW CALIBRATION MODEL

The basic modification which has been made to the previous calibration method is to plot, instead of PT ratios, the PTs themselves on logarithmic scales (Fig. 2). This has the advantage that the normal plasmas, as well as the patients' plasmas, appear explicitly as individual data points. The use of logarithmic scales, which are common in coagulation tests, has the advantage that the scatter in the data is then more uniform across the full range of times, and, as will be seen later, it also leads very naturally to a simple method of standardising PT ratios.

From empirical observation it appears that the relationship between the log PTs for two thromboplastins is either linear or very close to linear, even in cases where the Biggs-Denson model breaks down (8,9). The equation for the line is of the form

$$\log PT_v = c \log PT_h + d \qquad \text{(Equation 2)}$$

where c is the slope, d the intercept, and v and h signify the vertical and horizontal axes, respectively. Equation 2 forms the basis of the new WHO calibration scheme for thromboplastin calibration.

The calibration of a thromboplastin is defined by the slope, c, that is obtained when it is compared with a single reference preparation. The reference preparation is the International Reference Preparation (IRP) for Thromboplastin, Human, Combined (coded 67/40), which was established by the WHO Expert Committee on Biological Standardisation (11). When the IRP (67/40) is represented on the vertical axis and the thromboplastin being calibrated is represented on the horizontal axis, the slope c is

14

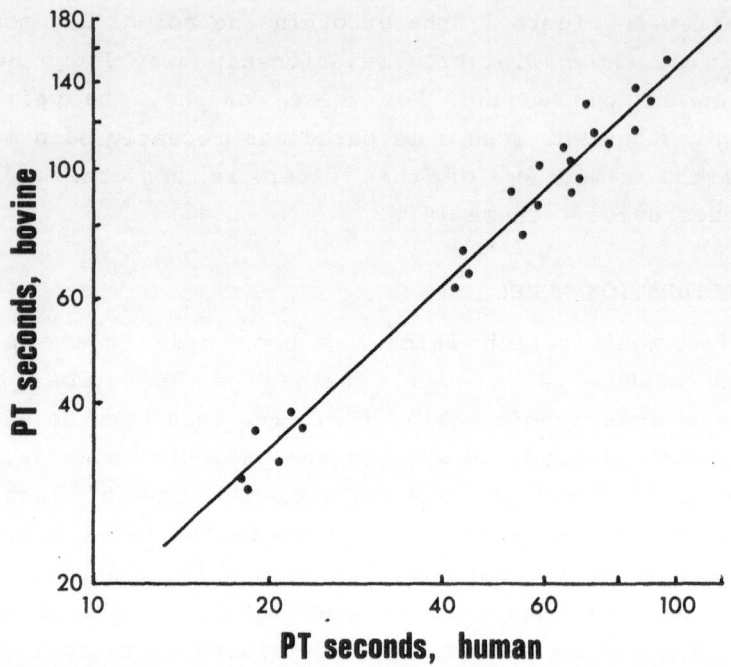

FIGURE 2. Log PT plot of data for 18 patients and 6 normals using a bovine thromboplastin (vertical axis) and a human thromboplastin (horizontal axis). The new WHO calibration procedure is based on fitting a straight line to all the data points (see Fig. 3).

defined as the International Sensitivity Index (ISI) of the latter preparation (see Fig. 3). In principle, any thromboplastin can thus be calibrated in terms of the primary IRP (67/40), although in practice it is common to use a secondary reference material as an intermediary (see below).

It should be remarked that the intercept, d, does not feature in the WHO calibration scheme because d is not needed in the standardisation of PT ratios (see next section), nor is it required for the serial calibration of one thromboplastin in terms of another which has already been assigned an ISI. For serial calibration all that is required is the multiplication of slopes. This has the fortunate consequence that only a single number, the ISI, is required to characterise the calibration process.

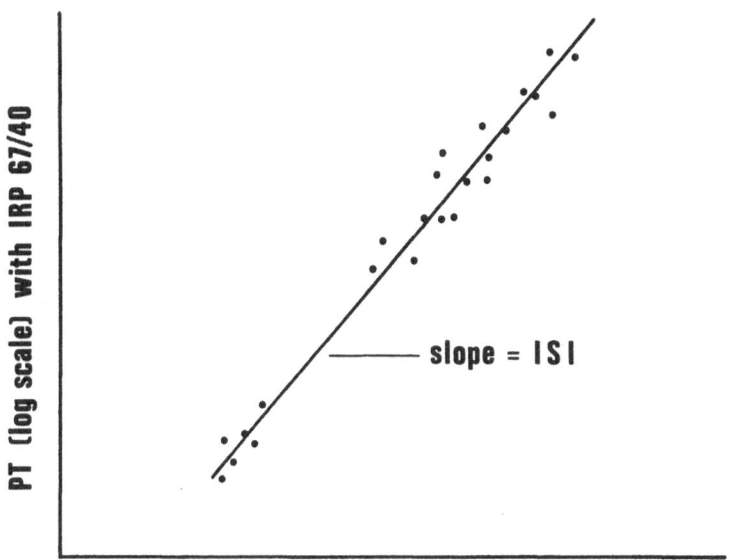

FIGURE 3. The International Sensitivity Index (ISI) of a thromboplastin is defined as the slope of the line in a log PT plot
where the thromboplastin represented on the vertical axis is the
primary human IRP (67/40). Calibration of an ISI may also be done
against a secondary reference thromboplastin, in which case the
ISI is obtained by multiplying the slope of the line by the ISI
for the secondary reference preparation (see text).

STANDARDISATION OF THE PT RATIO

From equation 2 a very simple relationship between the PT
ratios for the two thromboplastins can be derived (see Appendix).
This has the form

$$y = x^c \qquad\qquad \text{(Equation 3)}$$

where y and x are the PT ratios for the thromboplastins represented on the vertical and horizontal axes, respectively. To
convert a PT ratio for one thromboplastin into a PT ratio for
another, all that is required, therefore, is to know the slope in

the log PT plot. When the thromboplastin represented on the vertical axis is the IRP (67/40), so that c is the ISI of the other thromboplastin on the horizontal axis, the ratio y is defined as the International Normalised Ratio (INR). In other words, the equation INR = x^{ISI} gives the INR corresponding to any PT ratio x.

The INR defines the 'single scale' to which Biggs and Denson (2) aspired. For any thromboplastin, any measured PT ratio can be converted into an INR provided the ISI of the thromboplastin has previously been determined. The INR is, in effect, the scale on which the PT ratio of the patient in question would have been measured has the test been carried out using the IRP (67/40). The standardisation of PT ratios which is made possible through the use of thromboplastin calibration and INRs is thus equivalent to having all centres use the same thromboplastin, although it is much simpler to operate and it permits different centres to use in practice the thromboplastin which suits them best.

USE OF SECONDARY REFERENCE THROMBOPLASTINS

To determine the ISI of every thromboplastin by direct calibration against the primary IRP (67/40) would rapidly exhaust the stocks of the primary IRP. For this reason the WHO Expert Committee on Biological Standardisation (13) has recommended the use of secondary thromboplastin reference preparations which have been carefully calibrated against the primary material. In the calibration of a working thromboplastin against a secondary reference preparation, a calibration line in the form of equation 2 is determined, and the resulting slope c_{ws} is multiplied by the ISI of the secondary reference preparation, ISI_s, to give the ISI of the working thromboplastin $ISI_w = c_{ws} \times ISI_s$. By considering how c_{ws} and ISI_s are defined, it may readily be seen that apart from the extra statistical imprecision arising from the use of two calibration steps instead of one, ISI_w will be the same as if the working preparation had been calibrated directly against the primary IRP.

In keeping with the general principle of biological standardisation that like should preferably be compared with like, the WHO

Expert Committee on Biological Standardisation (13) recommends
that thromboplastins should as far as possible be calibrated
against reference preparations of the same species and to this
end it has established International Reference Preparations for
Bovine Thromboplastin (68/434) and for Rabbit Thromboplastin
(RBT/79) which have been calibrated against the primary human IRP
(67/40). The general system of thromboplastin calibration should
therefore operate as in Figure 4.

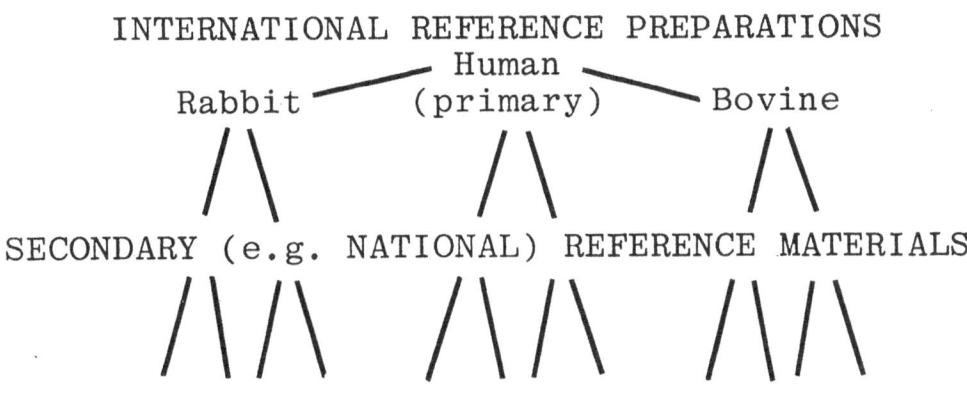

FIGURE 4. General scheme of thromboplastin calibration based on
the WHO International Reference Preparations.

In due course, even with the use of secondary reference thromboplastins, the primary IRP needs replacement, as is currently in
progress for 67/40, and this is done by calibrating the new primary IRP directly against the old one. When the original IRP
(67/40) is no longer available this will mean that the INR will
relate to a material which no longer exists, but this will not in

any way detract from the usefulness of the INR as a fully work-
able standardised scale.

HOW TO PERFORM A CALIBRATION STEP

The complexity of the calibration exercise will depend to a
large extent on the future role of the material which is to be
calibrated. For an international or national reference material a
multi-centre study is required so that (i) the calibration relationship can be validated with more than one test system, and
(ii) the magnitude of centre-to-centre variation in the calibration slope can be measured. A detailed account of the design and
analysis of a multi-centre calibration exercise can be found in
the report of the Bureau Communautaire de Référence calibration
of three certified reference materials for use among the member
nations of the EEC (5,9). For a material of lesser status it may
be sufficient to perform the calibration within a single centre.

In each case, the basic mode of calibration is to measure the
PTs for a set of patients' and normal plasmas using both the
reference thromboplastin and the material to be calibrated. These
are then used to plot a graph where the log PTs for the reference
preparation are represented on the vertical axis and the log PTs
for the material being calibrated are represented on the horizontal axis. A calibration line is then fitted to the resulting
data points. The statistical method of fitting the line is not
prescribed, but it is inappropriate to use ordinary least squares
regression since this leads to underestimation of the slope of
the true relationship when, as is the case with log PTs, the
variables on both axes are subject to random error and biological
variation. A recommended method is the technique of orthogonal
regression (9,10) in which the sum of squared deviations perpendicular to the regression line is minimised. Using orthogonal
regression it is also possible to calculate the standard error of
the calibration slope and, in the case where calibration is done
against a secondary reference preparation, this should be
combined with the standard error of the ISI of the secondary
reference preparation to give a composite standard error for the
ISI of the new material which takes into account the errors in

both calibration steps (13).

PT VERSUS PT RATIO

In some regions, standardisation schemes are already in operation which are based on standardising the PT, not the PT ratio. In the international scheme the WHO Expert Committee on Biological Standardisation, following Biggs and Denson (2), selected to standardise the PT ratio. The main reasons for this choice were, firstly, that the PT ratio is more robust than the PT against differences in experimental technique (6,14) and, secondly, that standardisation based on equation 3 requires only one number to be defined (the slope, or ISI), whereas standardisation based on equation 2 would require two (i.e., the intercept, d, as well). There is no reason, however, why PTs should not continue to be used locally in regions where the normal PT is demonstrably stable and effective standardisation of the PT test procedure is in operation as, for example, with the U.S. National Committee for Clinical Laboratory Standards procedural guidelines (4). Under these circumstances, however, it is a trivial matter to calculate PT ratios, and hence INRs as well, since PT and PT ratio differ only by a constant divisor.

DISCREPANCIES FROM THE CALIBRATION MODEL

Since the calibration model is an empirical representation of the relationship between thromboplastins, it is only to be expected that instances of discrepancy from equation 2 will occasionally arise. Such instances have, in fact, already been noted and are discussed in later papers in this volume. The question which must be decided in these cases is whether the discrepancy is large enough to require that some special account should be taken of it.

Firstly, it should be marked that not all statistically significant discrepancies are necessarily cause for alarm. A significant result can arise purely by chance, the meaning of significance at the 5% level being that a discrepancy as large as the one observed could be expected as a consequence solely of random variation in 5% of cases. Or, it may be that the discrepancy, although significant by statistical criteria, is nonetheless too small to matter. As in most other areas of biological standardisation it must be recognised that the complexities of biological reality will render any precise mathematical description a little inexact, and the ultimate criterion for the seriousness of a discrepancy from the model will be its likely effect on clinical practice. In general, it has been found that the new calibration model provides a very satisfactory description of the experimental results, and an advantage of the log PT plot showing the basic data for both the normal plasmas and the patients' plasmas is that in cases of discrepancy from the model the nature of the problem can readily be seen.

CONCLUSIONS

Using the WHO scheme for thromboplastin calibration any thromboplastin may be calibrated in terms of any other for its relative sensitivity to anticoagulant-induced prolongation of the prothrombin time and, in particular, each thromboplastin may be calibrated in terms of the primary IRP (67/40). The responsibility for calibrating new thromboplastins will usually rest with the manufacturers or with the national control authorities, although individual laboratories will also be able readily to calibrate working preparations for their own use. At present, the calibration relationship is defined only in terms of fresh plasmas, because it is required to represent tests as they are actually carried out on clinical samples, but it is possible that in future deep frozen or lyophilised plasma pools could be used both to reduce the total number of samples which are required and to permit a calibration to be made in circumstances where patients' plasmas are not readily available. Before pooled plasmas can be used with confidence, however, it must be demonstrated that the calibration relationship between the preparations is satisfactorily linear and that the pooled plasmas give PTs which lie on or near the straight line that best fits the data points for individual fresh samples.

Once a calibrated thromboplastin is available in the anti-coagulation clinic, it is a simple matter to calculate the INR for any given patient's plasma. Firstly, the mean PT for normal plasmas must be determined, the geometric mean being used in preference to the arithmetic mean (8) although the difference is not likely to be large. Secondly, the PT ratio, R, should be calculated. Thirdly, R should be converted into an INR using the equation $INR = R^{ISI}$. This conversion can be carried out in a few seconds on an inexpensive pocket calculator and, if the facility to calculate fractional powers is not available, the equivalent formula

$$INR = antilog (ISI \times log R)$$

can be used. Alternatively, a simple conversion table or chart can be prepared to avoid the need to use a calculator.

If medical staff and health auxiliaries involved in control-ling anticoagulant therapy become familiarised with the INR, as is urged by the World Health Organisation, then results and treatment policies specified in terms of INRs will be fully in-terchangeable between different centres using different working thromboplastins and will, furthermore, not require modification should one thromboplastin be replaced with another. When this state is attained, the goal set out by Biggs and Denson (2) will have been reached.

REFERENCES

1. Alderson MR, Poller L, Thomson JM. Validity of the British system for anticoagulant control using the national rea-gent. J Clin Pathol 1970; 23: 281-285.
2. Biggs R, Denson KWE. Standardisation of the one-stage pro-thrombin time for the control of anticoagulant therapy. Brit Med J 1967; 1: 84-88.
3. Exner T, Rickard KA, Kronenburg H. Comparison of throm-boplastin used for oral anticoagulant control. Pathology 1980; 12: 559-566.
4. Gralnick HR, Evatt BL, Huseby RM, Triplett DA. Procedural standards for the prothrombin time. In: Standardisation of Coagulation Assays: An Overview (ed. Triplett DA), College of American Pathologists, Skokie Illinois 1982; 51-55.
5. Hermans J. The European Community Bureau of Reference Cali-bration Study. This volume, Chapter 4.

6. ICTH/ICSH. Prothrombin time standardization: report of the expert panel on oral anticoagulant control. Thromb Haemostas 1979; 42: 1073-1114.
7. Kahan J, Noren I. Assessment of different mathematical models for calculating and expressing the results of coagulation test procedures. Thrombos Diathes Haemorrh 1975; 34: 522-530.
8. Kirkwood TBL. Calibration of reference thromboplastins and standardisation of the prothrombin time ratio. Thromb Haemostas 1983; 49: 238-244.
9. Loeliger EA, Van den Besselaar AMHP, Hermans J, Van der Velde EA. Certification of Three Reference Materials for Thromboplastins. BCR Information, Commission of the European Communities, Brussels 1981.
10. Van· der Velde EA. Orthogonal regression equation. This volume, chapter 3.
11. WHO Expert committee on Biological Standardisation. 28th Report. WHO Technical Report Series 610: 14-15 and 45-51. WHO, Geneva, 1977.
12. WHO Expert committee on Biological Standardisation. 31st Report. WHO Technical Report Series 658: 185-205. WHO, Geneva, 1981.
13. WHO Expert committee on Biological Standardisation. 33rd Report. WHO Technical Report Series, 687: 81-105. WHO Geneva, 1983.
14. Zucker S, Brosious E, Cooper GR. One-stage prothrombin time survey. Amer J Clin Pathol 1970; 53: 340-347.

APPENDIX

The calibration equation for PTs

$$\log PT_v = c \log PT_h + d$$

may be converted into an equation for PT ratios as follows.

Since the same calibration line describes both the normal and the patients' PTs, the normal PTs (NPTs) are also related as above. Thus, if y and x denote the PT ratios on the vertical and horizontal axes, respectively,

$$
\begin{aligned}
y &= PT_v/NPT_v \\
&= \text{antilog}(c \log PT_h + d)/\text{antilog}(c \log NPT_h + d) \\
&= \text{antilog}(c \log PT_h + d - c \log NPT_h - d) \\
&= \text{antilog}(c \log\{PT_h/NPT_h\}) \\
&= (PT_h/NPT_h)^c \\
&= x^c.
\end{aligned}
$$

Chapter 3:   ORTHOGONAL REGRESSION EQUATION

E.A. VAN DER VELDE

1. INTRODUCTION

Calibration of a new thromboplastin against an already calibrated one may be considered as a problem of determining the
relationship between two different quantifications of a coumarin-
induced coagulation defect. One quantification (say X) corresponds with the new thromboplastin, the other quantification (say
Y) corresponds with the already calibrated one. This chapter will
deal with situations where it may be assumed that X and Y are
linearly related, i.e. the relationship between X and Y may
satisfactorily be described by an equation of the form

$$Y = A + BX \qquad\qquad\qquad \text{(equation 1)}$$

In this chapter it will not be discussed whether X and Y should
be given in terms of a prothrombin time (PT) or in terms of a
transformation of the original PT, such as for example the
logarithm of the PT (log PT). In the contribution of Kirkwood [1]
the use of log PT is advocated, because a more satisfactory
straight line relationship is obtained by plotting PT's for
patients and normals individually on logarithmic axes. This
plotting procedure is equivalent with considering the relationship between the log PT's in a plot with linear axes. Although it
is not essential for understanding the theory to be presented in
this chapter the reader may from now on look at X and Y as the
logarithms of the PT's obtained with the new and the already
calibrated thromboplastin, respectively.

If two different points on the straight line describing the
relationship between X and Y could be determined exactly, it
would be no problem to calculate A and B. If the coordinates of
these two points are respectively $(X_1; Y_1)$ and $(X_2; Y_2)$ the

value of for example B is

$$B = \frac{Y_2 - Y_1}{X_2 - X_1}$$ (equation 2)

i.e. B is the number of units of increase in Y per unit increase in X.

Plots representing the observed individual results show however that the individual points are scattered about a straight line. As a consequence the underlying (linear) relationship between X and Y cannot be determined exactly from the observations. A fitting procedure which appropriately takes into account the structure of the data gives in such a case an estimate of the line representing the underlying relationship. The model describing the structure of the data of thromboplastin calibration experiments will be given in section 2. In section 3 two consequences of the use of an inappropriate fitting procedure for thromboplastin calibration are mentioned. In section 4 a fitting procedure is described which seems to be more relevant for thromboplastin calibration. The computational formulae are given in section 5. In that section also formulae are given for the estimation of the standard deviations of the slope and the intercept of the fitted line.

In section 6 a proposal is given for testing the hypothesis that the underlying relationship for patients' data is also valid for normals.

2. STATISTICAL MODEL

Assume that the relationship between X and Y can be described satisfactorily with an equation of the form $Y = A + BX$. For N individuals assessments of X and Y are made. Let $(X_i; Y_i)$ be the point on the line of relationship corresponding to the i-th individual ($i = 1, 2, \ldots, N$) and let $(x_i; y_i)$ be the result of the assessments (Fig. 1). It is assumed that, due to random fluctuations (including also genuine biological variability) the x_i and y_i deviate from X_i and Y_i respectively. These deviations (sometimes also called disturbances) will be denoted with δ_i and ε_i:

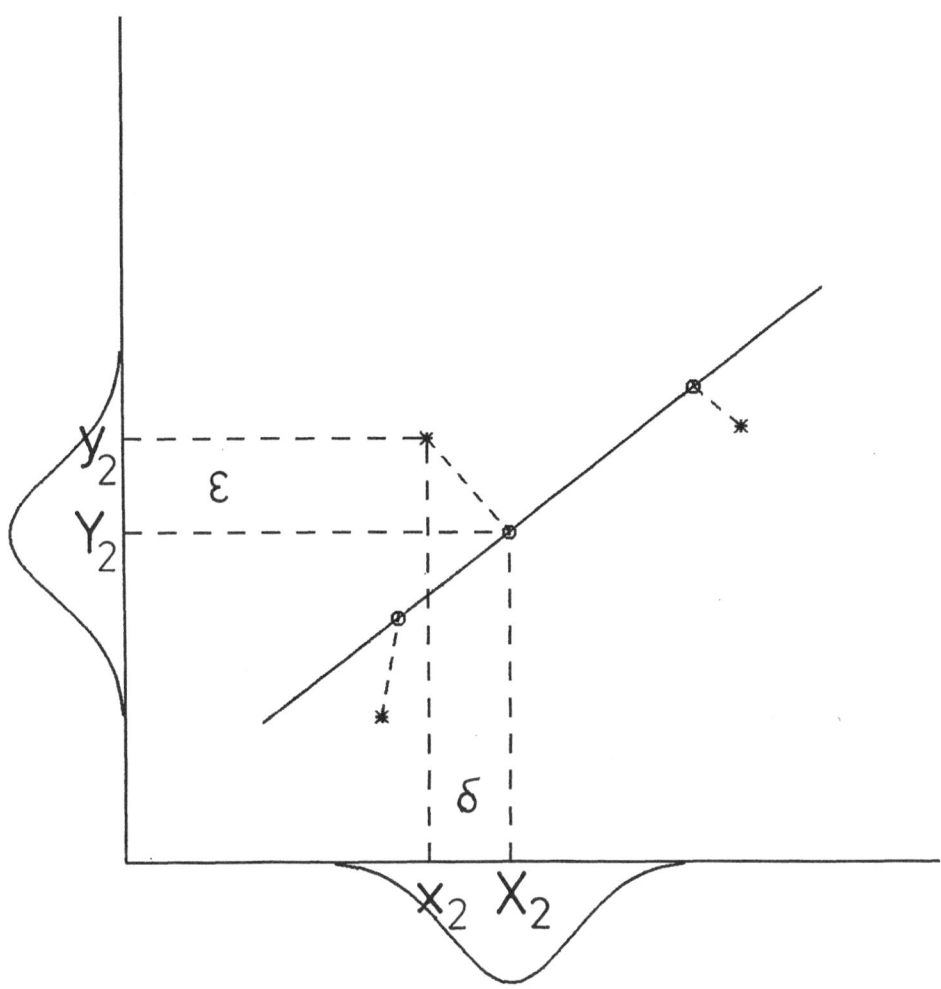

FIGURE 1. Model for a linear functional relationship with disturbances in both variables. Three points on the solid line (underlying relationship) are connected with the corresponding observed points (dotted lines). The normal frequency curves along the axes represent the distributions from which δ and ε (the distu..bances in x_2 and y_2) were randomly taken.

$$\delta_i = x_i - X_i \qquad \text{(equation 3)}$$

$$\varepsilon_i = y_i - Y_i \qquad \text{(equation 4)}$$

It is assumed that the δ's and ε's are mutually independent and normally distributed with zero means and standard deviations σ_δ (for all δ's) and σ_ε (for all ε's). By these assumptions the values $(X_i;Y_i)$ corresponding with points on the line $Y = A + BX$ are the expected values of $(x_i;y_i)$ which correspond with points about the line. The line $Y = A + BX$ is called the underlying line of relationship. In statistical literature a model as just described is often called a model for a functional relationship.

In the remainder of this chapter it is assumed that such a model gives a good description of the structure of the data obtained for the calibration of a new thromboplastin against an already calibrated thromboplastin.

It is noticed that the model is symmetric in x and y in the sense that in x as well as in y disturbances are supposed to be present. This is in contrast to the well-known regression model for linear relationships where for only one variable (say Y) the observations are supposed to be disturbed due to random fluctuations (ε_i) while the other variable (X) is known or observed without random deviations. This latter model is relevant for example in situations where one wants to calibrate an instrument for the determination of a (chemical) concentration. If in such a calibration experiment a number of solutions with known concentrations are assessed with the instrument, the known concentrations are the X's while the assessment obtained with the instrument are the y's. For the analysis of the data resulting from this type of experiment, the use of ordinary regression analysis may be appropriate. In the next section a short outline will be given of what happens if ordinary regression analysis would still be applied to thromboplastin calibration data where the more symmetric model for a functional relationship holds.

3. REGRESSION ANALYSIS IN THE CASE OF FUNCTIONAL RELATIONSHIP

Suppose that the functional relationship model of section 2 is relevant for the observations. Ordinary regression analysis only assumes random deviations in the Y-direction and neglects the fact that the observed points also deviate from the underlying line by random deviations in the X-direction. The line fitted to the data according to ordinary regression techniques minimizes the sum of squared distances in the Y-direction from the observed points to the line (see Fig. 2a). It can be proven that the slope (b) of this line tends to be smaller than the slope (B) of the underlying relationship. One can prove that for large numbers of individuals one has approximately:

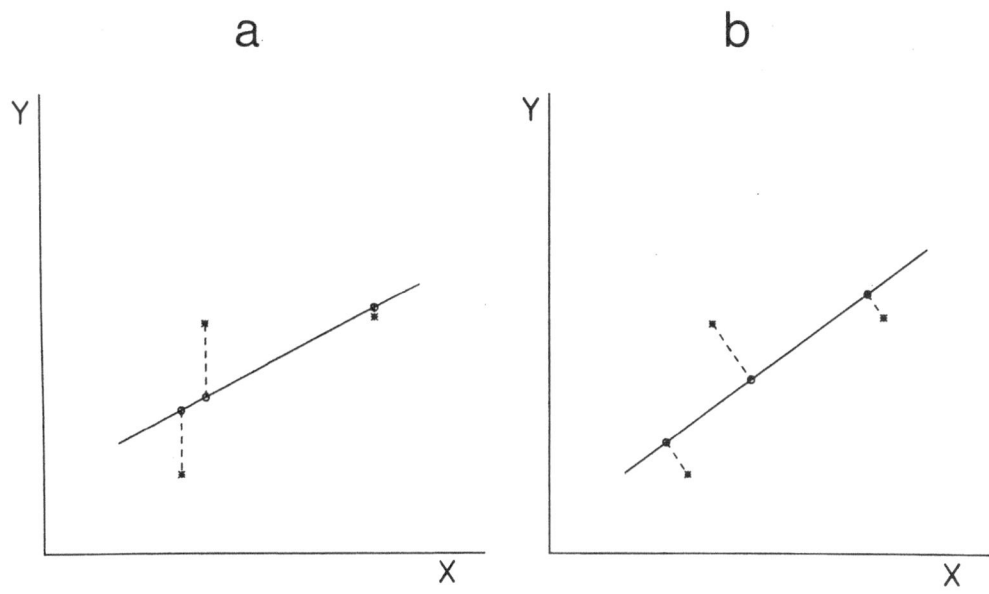

FIGURE 2. a) Ordinary regression line. The solid line minimizes the sum of squared distances of the observed points to the line. Distances are to be measured in the y-direction (dotted lines). b) Orthogonal regression line for the same observed points as presented in Fig. 2a. The sum of squared distances, measured in the direction orthogonal to the line, is now minimized.

$$b \sim \frac{s_X^2}{s_X^2 + \sigma_\delta^2} \cdot B = \frac{1}{1 + \sigma_\delta^2/s_X^2} \cdot B \qquad \text{(equation 5)}$$

with σ_δ as introduced in section 2 and

$$s_X^2 = \frac{\Sigma (X_i - \bar{X})^2}{N}$$

s_X may be considered as a measure for the extent to which the X-values are spread out. The factor with which B is multiplied in equation 5 equals 1 only if $\sigma_\delta/s_X = 0$, i.e. $\sigma_\delta = 0$, which is the case only if no disturbances are present in the X-direction. As soon as these disturbances are present the value of σ_δ becomes positive and the factor in equation 5 is smaller than 1. Regression analysis leads to an attenuated estimate of the slope B of the underlying line of relationship in cases where the functional relationship model is adequate ($\sigma_\delta > 0$). As on the one hand the value of σ_δ has in general a minimum which is inherent to the PT determination with the corresponding thromboplastin and on the other hand s_X is limited because of a limitation of the therapeutic range of anticoagulation intensity, the attenuation factor cannot be as close to 1 as one would wish. Notice also that an increase of the number of observations only reduces the variability of the slope of the regression line about the attenuated value but does not reduce the attenuation.

In a single calibration step the magnitude of the attenuation of the slope will in general not be dramatic. Two consequences of using the (inappropriate) regression analysis should, however, be mentioned.

1. According to the WHO proposal for calibrating a new thromboplastin patients as well as normals are to be assessed with both thromboplastins. As a first question then may arise: is the underlying relationship for the patients also valid for normals? Suppose that in a particular case this question should be answered affirmatively, i.e. the underlying line of relationship valid for patients' data coincides with that for normals' data. If for patients' data and normals' data separately regression

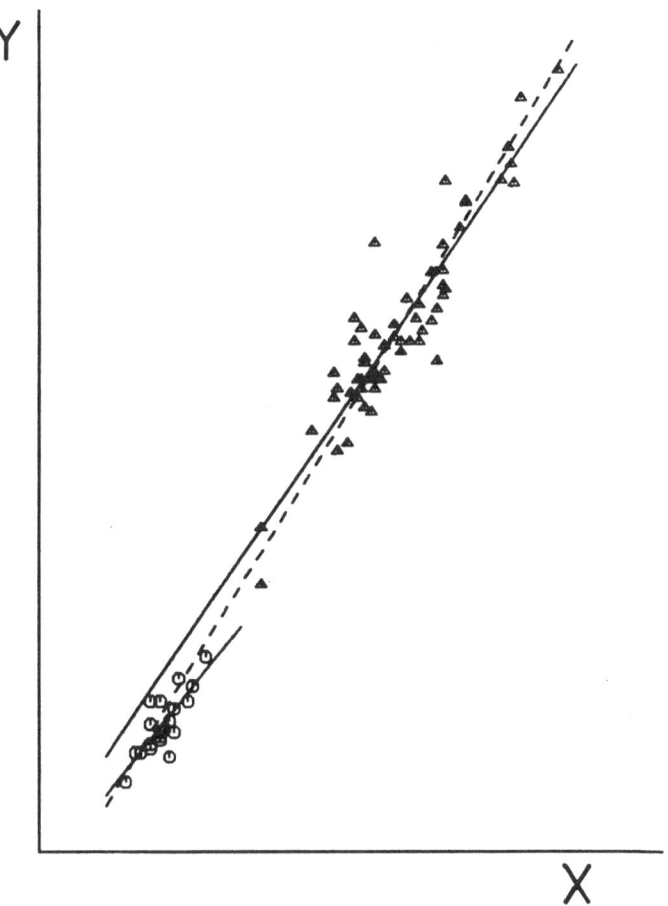

FIGURE 3. Regression lines may give misleading impressions. The data strongly suggest that the relationships of patients and normals coincide (dotted line), while the two regression lines (solid lines) are different due to attenuation.

lines are determined both lines will be attenuated and consequently the regression lines systematically tend to be different. As an illustration see Fig. 3 where clearly patients' data and normals' data can be described satisfactorily with one single straight line but where the regression line for patients' data differs from that for the normals' data. The dotted line in the figure is the orthogonal regression line obtained from the patients' data. This line will be introduced in section 4.

2. In the WHO scheme the final aim is to express the PT as found with the working thromboplastin in terms of some quantity defined on the scale of the International Reference Preparation (IRP) 67/40. This can be achieved by several intermediate calibration steps (for example: calibration of the working thromboplastin against a national reference preparation, which in turn has been calibrated against the International Reference Preparation). As the slope of the line of relationship between the working thromboplastin and the IRP 67/40 is obtained by multiplying the slopes of the calibration lines of the intermediate steps (1) the final result may seriously deviate from the slope which should have been obtained. Suppose for example that a working thromboplastin is calibrated and that there are two intermediate thromboplastins used. Let the attenuation factors in the intermediate steps be 0.97;0.93 and 0.95. Then the total attenuation is the product of these factors that is 0.86 which means that the final product slope is underestimated by 14%. Note again that these attenuations are not depending on N and thus that increasing the number of observations does not lead to a way out of this problem.

4. ORTHOGONAL REGRESSION

In section 2 the model describing the data for thromboplastin calibration was given. In section 3 it was shown that ordinary regression analysis by not taking into account the appropriate structure of the random fluctuations in the data leads to incorrect estimates even in the case of large numbers of observations. Unfortunately no good estimation procedure is possible unless an additional assumption is made. The additional assumption which is often made and also made in the remainder of this chapter is that $\sigma_\delta = \sigma_\epsilon$ (see section 2) i.e. the standard deviations of the disturbances are the same in the two directions X and Y. If this additional assumption is made, maximum likelihood estimates a and b of the parameters A and B of the underlying line of relationship exist. For a more detailed discussion, see Kendall and Stuart (2). The line which corresponds to these estimates a and b is the line which minimizes the sum of squared distances of the observed points to the line. These distances are to be measured in a direction orthogonal (perpendicular) to the line (see Fig. 2b). It can be shown that if the assumptions in the model (including $\sigma_\delta = \sigma_\varepsilon$) are fulfilled that the slope of the line thus obtained is not attenuated. For increasing numbers of observations (provided that s_X, the spread-out of the points, does not converge to zero) the difference between the fitted line and the line of the underlying relationship tends to disappear. Expressed in a more statistical-theoretical termi-nology: the orthogonal regression line estimates the underlying relationship consistently.

The deviation of the fitted line from the underlying relation-ship is due to random fluctuations δ_i and ε_i (equations 2 and 3). The standard deviation σ_ε (and also σ_δ which is supposed to be equal to σ_ε) can be estimated as follows. Suppose that an orthogonal regression line is fitted to the observed points and let the minimized sum of squared orthogonal distances to this line be denoted by SS. Then σ_δ and σ_ε are estimated by:

$$s = \left[SS/(N - 2) \right]^{\frac{1}{2}} \qquad \text{(equation 6)}$$

Quantity s is sometimes also called the standard deviation about the orthogonal regression line. In section 5 formulae are given for the computation of a, b and s for a given set of data. In addition estimates of the standard deviations of a and b are given. With these latter standard deviations one can estimate the precision of the orthogonal regression line.

In 1878 Adcock (3) recommended the use of the orthogonal regression line when uncorrected disturbances with equal variances are present in the observations of both variables. In 1979 the necessity for using a technique of this type rather than ordinary regression analysis was obviously not generally recog-nized: Cornbleet and Gochman (4) devoted a paper to essentially the same subject. The reluctance of many investigators to use something different from ordinary regression analysis might be related i.a. to the absence of computational facilities on

computers for the calculation of an orthogonal regression line
and measures of variability such as standard deviation about the
line and the precision of the line. Indeed, formulae for the
calculation of the precision of the orthogonal regression line
remained unknown for quite a long time. It is remarkable that in
1979 Patefield (5) not only reported the correct formulae for the
estimation of the variances and covariance of a and b of the
orthogonal regression line, but also criticized two earlier
(although recent) publications in which inconsistent estimators
of these (co)variances were given.

5. COMPUTATIONAL FORMULAE

Let the data consist of N pairs of observations with
$(x_i; y_i)$ denoting the pair corresponding to the i-th individual. Suppose that the model of a functional relationship as
described in section 2 with the additional assumption $\sigma_\delta = \sigma_\varepsilon$
is relevant for the data. The following notations will be used:

$$\bar{x} = (\Sigma x)/N \qquad\qquad \bar{y} = (\Sigma y)/N \qquad \text{(equations 7a, 7b)}$$

$$S_{xx} = \Sigma (x - \bar{x})^2 \qquad\qquad S_{yy} = \Sigma (y - \bar{y})^2 \qquad \text{(equations 7c, 7d)}$$

$$S_{xy} = \Sigma (x - \bar{x})(y - \bar{y}) \qquad\qquad \text{(equation 7e)}$$

The reader is supposed to be familiar with the use of the Σ-sign
to denote a summation. For example:

$$\Sigma xy = x_1 y_1 + x_2 y_2 + \cdots x_N y_N$$

The slope b and the intercept a of the orthogonal regression line
are:

$$b = \frac{S_{yy} - S_{xx} + \left[(S_{yy} - S_{xx})^2 + 4S_{xy}^2\right]^{\frac{1}{2}}}{2S_{xy}} \qquad \text{(equation 8)}$$

$$a = \bar{y} - b\bar{x} \qquad\qquad \text{(equation 9)}$$

The minimized sum of squared orthogonal distances of the observed points to the fitted line can be computed by:

$$SS = S_{yy} - bS_{xy} \qquad \text{(equation 10)}$$

The estimate s of the common value of σ_δ and σ_ε is thus (cf. equation 6):

$$s = [SS/(N-2)]^{\frac{1}{2}} = [(S_{yy} - bS_{xy})/(N-2)]^{\frac{1}{2}} \qquad \text{(equation 11)}$$

The standard deviation of b can be estimated by

$$s_b = \left[\frac{\{(1+b^2)s_{xy} + s^2b\}s^2b}{Ns_{xy}^2} \right]^{\frac{1}{2}} \qquad \text{(equation 12)}$$

with $s_{xy} = S_{xy}/N$

The standard deviation of a can be estimated with

$$s_a = \left[\frac{(1 + b^2)s^2}{N} + \bar{x}^2 s_b^2 \right]^{\frac{1}{2}} \qquad \text{(equation 13)}$$

Let Y_0 be the value of the variable Y which corresponds according to the underlying relationship with a given value X_0 of the variable X. So $Y_0 = A + BX_0$. For the given value X_0, the value Y_0 is estimated by $y_0 = a + bX_0$, where b and a are obtained from equations 8 and 9. The standard deviation of y_0 can be estimated with:

$$s_{y_0} = \left[\frac{(1 + b^2)s^2}{N} + (\bar{x} - X_0)^2 s_b^2 \right]^{\frac{1}{2}} \qquad \text{(equation 14)}$$

which for the special choice of $X_0 = 0$ is reduced to equation 13.

Patefield (5) gave an estimate of the covariance matrix of a and b. Equations 12 and 13 are in fact his results in a different notation. Equation 14 can easily be derived from his results.

For the actual computations some simplifications can be made. The computation of S_{xx}, S_{yy} and S_{xy} can be simplified with the well-known reduction formulae:

$$S_{xy} = \Sigma xy - N\bar{x}\bar{y}$$

$$S_{xx} = \Sigma x^2 - N\bar{x}^2$$

$$S_{yy} = \Sigma y^2 - N\bar{y}^2$$

If a pocket calculator is available with statistical functions built in, one can enter the pairs of observations according to the instructions in the manual for a regression problem. Then $S_{xx} = (N-1)s_x^2$, $S_{yy} = (N-1)s_y^2$ and $S_{xy} = (N-1)rs_x s_y$, where s_x and s_y are the standard deviations of x and y and r is the correlation coefficient of x and y. The manual of the calculator must give instructions how to obtain the values of these latter three statistics.

Provided that r>0, equation 8 can also be written as:

$$b = m + \left[m^2 + 1\right]^{\frac{1}{2}} \qquad \text{(equation 15)}$$

with $m = \dfrac{1}{2r} \left[\dfrac{s_y}{s_x} - \dfrac{s_x}{s_y}\right]$

Likewise, equation 11 can be rewritten as:

$$s = \left[\frac{N-1}{N-2} \cdot \left[s_y^2 - brs_x s_y\right]\right]^{\frac{1}{2}} \qquad \text{(equation 16)}$$

6. COMPARISON OF ORTHOGONAL REGRESSION LINES

In generally accessible statistical textbooks, hardly any attention seems to be given to the comparison of two or more functional relationships. In this section a technique will be suggested which will be explained intuitively.

Suppose first that the two underlying lines of relationship (one for the patients and one for the normals) are not coincident. In that case one single line can not be fitted to the pooled set of data equally well as two separate lines, one for each set. The minimized sum of squared distances of the pooled set of data to a common line tends to be (substantially) larger than the sum of squared distances which is obtained by fitting two lines which minimize the sum for each set separately. Let

SS_0 denote the outcome of equation 10, which is obtained for the pooled set of patients' and normals' data and let SS_N and SS_P denote the outcomes of equation 10 applied to the two sets separately. In case the underlying relationships are not coincident, SS_0 will be essentially larger than SS_N+SS_P. If on the other hand the two underlying relationships are coincident, then one line can in principle be fitted to the data equally well as two lines, one for each set separately. In this latter case SS_0 is not essentially larger than SS_N+SS_P (for numerical reasons SS_0 is never smaller than SS_N+SS_P). To decide whether the data contradict the hypothesis of coincidence of the underlying relationships, one might thus look at the relative degree with which SS_0 exceeds SS_N+SS_P. The following statistic is suggested:

$$F = \frac{SS_0 - (SS_N + SS_P)}{(SS_N + SS_P)} \cdot \frac{(N - 4)}{2} \qquad \text{(equation 17)}$$

where N is the total number of individuals (patients and normals). The factor $(N-4)/2$ in equation 17 is in analogy to the analysis of covariance.

Non-coincidence of two lines of linear relationship may be caused by two reasons: 1) the slopes are different (in that case there is in general no sense in investigating the equality of intercepts), or 2) the slopes are equal but the intercepts are not. To investigate especially whether the underlying lines are different because of non-parallelism, the same line of thought as presented above may be followed. However, in this case instead of one line, a pair of parallel lines is fitted to the data (one line for the patients, the other for the normals) such that the sum of squared distances of the points to the corresponding line is minimized. The (common) slope of this pair of parallel lines and the total sum of squared distances is obtained by applying equations 8 and 10 to SS_{xx}, S_{yy} and S_{xy} which are obtained as follows:

$$S_{xx} = (S_{xx})_{pat} + (S_{xx})_{norm}$$

$$S_{yy} = (S_{yy})_{pat} + (S_{yy})_{norm}$$

$$S_{xy} = (S_{xy})_{pat} + (S_{xy})_{norm}$$

where the terms in the right-hand sides of these equations are obtained in an obvious way by application of equations 7 to the patients' and normals' data separately. Let SS_0' be the thus obtained outcome of equation 10 for the parallel lines. Then for testing the hypothesis of parallelism of the underlying relationships one might use:

$$F_P = \frac{SS_0' - (SS_P + SS_N)}{SS_P + SS_N} \cdot \frac{(N - 4)}{1} \qquad \text{(equation 18)}$$

If one assumes parallelism, the hypothesis of equal intercepts can be investigated with

$$F_C = \frac{SS_0 - SS_0'}{SS_P + SS_N} \cdot \frac{(N - 4)}{1} \qquad \text{(equation 19)}$$

The distributions of F_P and F_C are very complicated. However, analogously to the analysis of covariance to be used for the comparison of regression lines, one might expect that under the respective null-hypotheses F_P and F_C follow approximately an F-distribution with 1 and N-4 degrees of freedom. Monte Carlo experiments showed that for F_C this approximation is very satisfactory for all settings of the common slope and σ_δ ($=\sigma_\varepsilon$), which are relevant for thromboplastin calibration problems.

It also turned out that the statistic F_P does not follow the F-distribution in a quite satisfactory way. The type I error turned out to be larger than claimed, i.e. the null-hypothesis of parallelism is rejected too often.

Fortunately, in thromboplastin calibration problems the test for parallelism is not as important as the test for coincidence. As the range of PT values of the normals is substantially smaller than that of the patients, the test based on F_C may be used to investigate whether the mean values of the normals are on the patients' line, even if the relationships of normals and patients are not quite parallel. The use of F_C (equation 19) is preferred to that of F (equation 17) because F was found to have the same drawbacks as F_P (equation 18) in the Monte Carlo experiments.

REFERENCES

1. Kirkwood TBL. General aspects of thromboplastin calibration. This volume, chapter 2.
2. Kendall MG, Stuart A. The advanced theory of statistics, 3rd edition. Griffin, London 1973. Vol. 2, chapter 29: pp. 375-418.
3. Adcock RJ. A problem in least squares. Analyst 1878; 5: 53-55.
4. Cornbleet PJ, Gochman N. Incorrect least-squares regression coefficients in method comparison analysis. Clin Chem 1979; 25: 432-438.
5. Patefield WM. On the information matrix in the linear functional relationship problem. Applied Statistics 1977; 26: 69-70.

Chapter 4:   THE   EUROPEAN   COMMUNITY   BUREAU   OF   REFERENCE
             CALIBRATION STUDY*

J. HERMANS

1. INTRODUCTION

Monitoring of oral anticoagulation is done on the basis of the results of a coagulation time determination in patient blood (or plasma), called the prothrombin time (PT) test. This test requires tissue extracts called thromboplastins. Tissue sources are usually rabbit brain, rabbit lung, human brain, or ox brain. Thromboplastins from different sources lead to quite different levels of prothrombin times. This points to the need for conversion of these prothrombin times to a common scale.

To make possible such a conversion, three reference thromboplastins were laid down several years ago in a joint effort of the International Committee on Thrombosis and Haemostasis (ICTH) and the World Health Organisation (WHO). They were representatives of the three major brain tissue types used at present: human (67/40), bovine (68/434) and rabbit (70/178). The human thromboplastin was designated as the primary reference preparation. The other two thromboplastins are secondary reference preparations. The secondaries were calibrated against the primary, and it was required that any other thromboplastin be calibrated against the reference of its own type.

---

*This paper is very similar to the paper 'A Collaborative Calibration Study of Reference Materials for Thromboplastins' by J. Hermans, A.M.H.P. van den Besselaa·, E.A. Loeliger and E.A. van der Velde, Thromb Haemostas (Stuttgart, 1983; 50(3):712-717. Kind permission of the publisher of Thrombosis and Haemostasis, F.K. Schattauer Verlag GmbH, was obtained.

The method of calibration adopted by WHO/ICTH (1,2) was suggested by Biggs and Denson (3). They considered the prothrombin time ratio, i.e. a patient's prothrombin time (PT) divided by the average PT for normal plasma. Biggs and Denson observed that if for a set of patient's plasmas the PT ratios obtained with two different thromboplastins are plotted against one another an approximately straight line is obtained. This line with its single parameter, the slope as the calibration constant was used for calibration purpose until 1982 (4).

A re-examination of the methodology for calibrating one thromboplastin against another led to an alternative approach. Basically, this approach starts with plotting, not PT ratios for patients but the PTs themselves for patients and normals on a logarithmic scale. A detailed discussion on the arguments for proposing this alternative method for calibrating thromboplastins, is given by Kirkwood (5). A summary of the method will be given under Materials and Methods.

A practical problem is that the reference thromboplastins of course exist only in finite supply and are at the disposal of national reference laboratories only. To enable manufacturers to relate their materials more easily to the WHO reference, three candidate reference thromboplastins have been developed in a joint effort of the International Committee for Standardization in Haematology (ICSH) and the Community Bureau of Reference (BCR) of the European Communities. Again, each of the three major brain tissues is represented: human (BCT/099), ox/bovine (OBT/79), and rabbit (RBT/79). These three candidate reference thromboplastins as well as the three WHO reference preparations have been used in the collaborative study reported here. Detailed information is given under Materials and Methods.

The present paper contains the results obtained by ten (seven European and three American) laboratories. It gives results of relating the secondary international reference preparations (68/434, 70/178) and the new candidate reference preparations (BCT/099, OBT/79, and RBT/79) to the primary international reference thromboplastin (67/40).

For the seven European laboratories a workshop was organized before starting the study, in order to test the protocol in all details. The American laboratories could not attend this workshop. The results of the seven European laboratories with respect to the three candidate reference thromboplastins, formed the basis of the BCR certification and they are described in a BCR report (6). The present paper reports and summarizes the calibration results of these seven European laboratories for all five thromboplastins. The results of the three American laboratories will be considered for confirmation purposes.

2. MATERIALS AND METHODS

2.1. Reference materials

Table 1 Characteristics of thromboplastin reference materials

	Codes Reference Materials WHO 67/40	68/434	70/178	BCR BCT/099	OBT/79	RBT/79
Brain tissue type	human	bovine	rabbit	human	bovine	rabbit
Plain/combined[1]	combined	combined	plain	plain	combined	plain
Vials/ampoules	sealed glass ampoules	sealed glass ampoules	sealed glass ampoules	rubber-capped vials	sealed glass ampoules	sealed glass ampoules
Initial mass or volume ($\pm$ sd)	2.051 $\pm$ 0.025 g	2.2 $\pm$ 0.01 g	1.029 $\pm$ 0.01 g	1.45 $\pm$ 0.03 g	2.211 $\pm$ 0.005 g	0.5 $\pm$ 0.02 ml
Gaseous phase	nitrogen	vacuum	nitrogen	vacuum	vacuum	nitrogen (86.7 KPa)
Water mass fraction after lyophilization (kg/kg)	0.0064	0.021	0.0069	<0.02	0.016	<0.01
To be reconstituted with	2.0 ml CaCl$_2$ (3.2 mmol/l)	2.2 ml CaCl$_2$ (3.2 mmol/l)	1.0 ml distilled water	1.0 ml water+ phenol (0.5 g/l)	2.2 ml CaCl$_2$ (3.2 mmol/l)	0.5 ml distilled water
pH				6.5	7.73	6.8
Haemoglobin				b.d.l.[2]	b.d.l.[2]	b.d.l.[2]

[1] also contains fibrinogen and coagulation Factor V
[2] below detection limit

The main characteristics of the six reference materials are summarized in Table 1. The WHO materials are stored at the National Institute for Biological Standards and Control (NIBSC) in London, U.K.; the BCR materials at the National Institute of Public Health (RIV) at Bilthoven, The Netherlands. The three BCR reference materials are:

- a lyophilized batch of British Comparative Thromboplastin (BCT/099) prepared by courtesy of Dr. L. Poller, Manchester, U.K.;
- a bovine type (OBT/79) prepared by courtesy of Nyegaard & Co., Oslo, Norway;
- a rabbit type (RBT/79) prepared by courtesy of Dr. K.W.E. Denson, Thame, U.K.

2.2 Experimental Procedures for Calibration

The calibration study was performed in accordance with an extensive protocol. A summary of the protocol is given here; the full protocol is given in Annex I, pp. 60-76.

Results were obtained from ten different laboratories in order to assess the inter-laboratory variation. To include the effect of inter-day variation, prothrombin time determinations were performed in each laboratory on at least six and preferably ten different days. On each day each laboratory had to include two freshly prepared "normal" specimens and six freshly prepared patient specimens. Normals were recruited from the laboratory staff. Patients had to have been stabilized on anti-coagulation; the criterion for "stabilized" was considered to be a prothrombin time with 67/40 between 1.5 and 5 times the mean "normal" 67/40 time, for at least 6 weeks. On each day a different set of eight subjects was taken. All coagulation endpoints were read visually with the tilt-tube technique. Actual testing was performed such that for each subject all six thromboplastins were used consecutively; after that the same procedure was followed for the next subject. The testing order of the subjects was the same as their order of blood sampling. The order of thromboplastins on each day was varied as prescribed in the protocol. For all other technical details the protocol should be consulted.

2.3. Statistical procedures

For reasons outlined in (5) it is preferred to relate the logarithms of the prothrombin times for the two thromboplastins. The relationship between the two thromboplastins in the log PT

plot appeared to be linear or very close to linear (see Results).
So its equation is of the form

$$y = a + bx \qquad \text{(equation 1)}$$

where a is the intercept, b is the slope, and x and y denote log
PTs. Since the primary reference 67/40 defines the common scale
to which the other thromboplastins have to be converted, it is
convenient for the plot and equation 1 to take 67/40 for the
vertical axis (y) and the secondary thromboplastins for the horizontal axis (x). Calibration equation 1 is characterized by two
parameters; having determined these parameters for some secondary
thromboplastin a prothrombin time with this thromboplastin is
then straightforwardly converted to the common scale of the 67/40
thromboplastin.

If one and the same calibration equation y=a+bx is valid for
both patients and normals it is moreover easily possible, using
only the slope b, to convert a prothrombin time ratio from one
thromboplastin to another. It can be shown, see (5), that under
the above mentioned condition (the same calibration equation for
patients and normals)

$$R_{67/40} = R_{RM}^{b} \qquad \text{(equation 2)}$$

where $R_{67/40}$ and R_{RM} are the prothrombin time ratios for
67/40 and another reference material (RM), respectively, and b is
the slope of the calibration line in equation 1. Ratios converted
to the scale of 67/40 are termed <u>international normalized ratios</u>,
and slope b is called the <u>international sensitivity index</u> (7).

The next item of statistical concern is how to estimate the
parameters a and b of the calibration equation 1. As is well
known from the clinical-chemistry literature, e.g. (8), the ordinary least squares linear regression equations to estimate slope
(a) and intercept (b) are not appropriate when both sets of measurements are subject to error. A more versatile method to estimate slope and intercept is the technique of <u>orthogonal</u> regression. This technique minimizes the squared deviations in the
direction perpendicular to the fitted line. The method handles

both sets of measurements in a fully symmetric way. Its estimates of slope and intercept are

$$b = m + \left[m^2 + 1\right]^{\frac{1}{2}} \qquad \text{(equation 3a)}$$

$$m = \frac{\Sigma(y-\bar{y})^2 - \Sigma(x-\bar{x})^2}{2\Sigma(x-\bar{x})(y-\bar{y})} = \frac{1}{2r}\left[\frac{S_y}{S_x} - \frac{S_x}{S_y}\right] \qquad \text{(equation 3b)}$$

and $a = \bar{y} - b\bar{x}$ (equation 3c)

(r=coefficient of correlation; S_x and S_y are the standard deviations of x and y, and $\bar{y}$ and $\bar{x}$ are the mean values of y and x, respectively). Measures for the variability are the standard deviation about the regression line and the standard errors of slope b and intercept a. The latter two are given in (9); see also (6). By modification of the statistical inference techniques of ordinary regression, procedures appropriate for orthogonal regressions such as estimates of precision, test of linearity, and test for coincidence of several lines, can be derived (see 10).

Implicit in the equations 3a and b is an assumption that the statistical errors on both axes are similar in magnitude. This cannot be tested on our data since they include both biological and experimental variations and the former cannot be reproduced easily. However, similarity of the two errors seems reasonable a priori and moreover the result is only marginally affected if the assumption is not strictly fulfilled. Should subsequent results reveal gross invalidity of this assumption, the equations 3a and b should be modified accordingly; a factor representing the ratio of the statistical errors then enters into the equations 3a and b.

3. RESULTS
3.1. Calibration results

All data submitted by the different laboratories to the department of Medical Statistics of the Leiden University are given in Annex 2, pp. 77-86.

Table 2 The number of days, normals, patients and exclusions for each laboratory

Lab	Number of days	Number of normals	Number of patients	Number of excluded specimen	Final total number of plasmas
1	10	20	60	4	76
2	10	18[1])	60	6	72
3	10	20	60	1	79
4	7	14	42	9	47
5	6	12	36	4	44
6	10	20	60	11	69
7	10	20	60	3	77
8	5	10	30	10	30
9	6	12	35	11	36
10	6	12	34	12	34
Total		158	477	71	564

[1]) Two missing observations due to technical failures

Table 2 gives for each laboratory (European 1-7, American 8-10) the number of plasmas used in the final analysis.

The 71 excluded specimens concerned in 68 cases patients whose 67/40 time was <1.5 or >5.0 times the mean of 67/40 time of the normals of the corresponding laboratory. Three of the 71 specimens were excluded because of outlying 67/40 times: one for lab 8 and two for lab 9. Outlying was defined by being outside the region defined by the orthogonal regression line ± 3 times the standard deviation around regression (calculated including all observations). In accordance with the same outlier criterion for nine specimens an observation for only one of the other thromboplastins had to be removed: three BCT/099, five OBT/79, and one 68/434.

Table 3 The means and standard deviations of the prothrombin times of the normal subjects for each laboratory given as time/s

Thromboplastin		67/40		68/434		70/178		BCT/099		OBT/79		RBT/79	
Lab	N	$\bar{x}$	s	$\bar{x}$	s	$\bar{x}$	s	$\bar{x}$	s	$\bar{x}$	s	$\bar{x}$	s
1	20	17.13	0.92	40.95	4.24	13.82	0.70	12.99	0.77	36.02	3.50	14.63	0.89
2	18	16.69	1.21	38.10	3.05	15.08	0.80	13.58	0.94	33.10	2.30	16.33	1.08
3	20	18.62	0.92	41.52	2.42	16.95	0.82	15.17	0.64	36.48	2.06	17.37	0.70
4	14	17.23	0.93	38.86	3.73	16.11	0.74	14.99	0.80	34.08	2.90	16.77	0.71
5	12	16.98	1.15	40.63	4.89	15.77	1.25	13.87	1.00	34.54	2.74	16.25	1.32
6	20	19.22	1.50	45.20	4.85	17.53	1.42	15.64	1.19	39.07	3.59	18.45	1.62
7	20	18.47	2.29	43.48	4.68	15.64	1.30	14.36	1.28	37.60	3.96	16.16	1.42
8	10	17.95	1.19	39.53	3.12	15.71	1.27	13.69	0.69	34.79	2.56	16.14	1.15
9	11	18.65	1.14	40.64	4.55	16.92	1.17	15.24	1.28	36.80	2.70	18.00	0.82
10	12	17.48	1.12	41.76	4.56	15.76	1.15	14.53	1.33	35.73	2.95	16.78	1.57

48

Table 3 summarizes the data of the normals. For each of the six thromboplastins the differences between the ten laboratories are highly significant (analysis of variance, p<0.01), so the laboratories have different levels for the mean normal time.

Relating the log seconds for each of the five thromboplastins to those of the primary reference 67/40, one has to investigate whether this relation* is the same for patients and normals. This comes down to examining whether two orthogonal regression lines (one for patients and one for normals) coincide. This examination showed statistical differences between the two lines more often than could be expected due to chance (see (6), Chapter 8.3.3). Clear examples of non-coincident lines are shown in Fig. 1. The pattern of Fig. 1 shows, however, that the line based on patients crosses the scatter of the normals. The line based on normals does not cross the patients' data, but, because of the much wider range of the patients' data (and therefore greater reliability of this line) we felt it justified to describe the relationship by one line based on the combined patients' and normals' data. The same argument held for the other cases of non-coinciding lines.

Table 4 Orthogonal regression equations y = a + bx for BCT/099, OBT/79, RBT/79, 68/434, and 70/178, respectively, (x-axis) versus 67/40 (y-axis). Data are in log (time/s). Tabulated are intercept I, slope b, standard error of the slope s (b) and standard deviation about the orthogonal regression line s. The intercepts I are at an x-value in the middle of the therapeutic range

	N	Human BCT/099 I = a+b·1.6	b	s (b)	s	Bovine OBT/79 I = a+b·2.0	b	s (b)	s	Rabbit RBT/79 I = a+b·1.5	b	s (b)	s
Lab 1	76	1.780	1.104	0.019	0.021	1.673	0.979	0.015	0.020	1.736	1.482	0.036	0.025
Lab 2	72	1.702	1.018	0.021	0.022	1.685	0.968	0.018	0.021	1.602	1.317	0.036	0.025
Lab 3	79	1.713	1.049	0.014	0.019	1.707	1.000	0.009	0.013	1.689	1.591	0.028	0.020
Lab 4	47	1.704	1.089	0.028	0.026	1.707	1.004	0.015	0.016	1.619	1.374	0.047	0.030
Lab 5	44	1.695	1.005	0.023	0.025	1.691	0.993	0.021	0.022	1.624	1.330	0.041	0.028
Lab 6	69	1.693	1.004	0.023	0.033	1.721	1.061	0.014	0.019	1.615	1.374	0.041	0.036
Lab 7	77	1.737	1.064	0.017	0.022	1.721	1.073	0.017	0.021	1.680	1.423	0.037	0.030
Lab 8	30	1.706	0.980	0.022	0.024	1.709	0.990	0.012	0.013	1.631	1.300	0.027	0.018
Lab 9	36	1.716	1.051	0.024	0.019	1.699	0.989	0.026	0.025	1.617	1.415	0.053	0.029
Lab 10	34	1.680	0.976	0.028	0.027	1.648	0.907	0.016	0.018	1.633	1.399	0.052	0.028

	N	68/434 I = a+b·2.0	b	s (b)	s	70/178 I = a+b·1.5	b	s (b)	s
Lab 1	76	1.636	1.023	0.019	0.024	1.837	1.668	0.033	0.019
Lab 2	72	1.631	0.979	0.022	0.025	1.699	1.486	0.046	0.026
Lab 3	79	1.658	1.019	0.012	0.017	1.744	1.729	0.035	0.021
Lab 4	47	1.645	0.994	0.019	0.020	1.701	1.599	0.048	0.024
Lab 5	44	1.625	1.006	0.031	0.033	1.727	1.623	0.054	0.026
Lab 6	69	1.665	1.091	0.018	0.022	1.702	1.620	0.048	0.032
Lab 7	77	1.653	1.078	0.025	0.031	1.745	1.593	0.042	0.028
Lab 8	30	1.659	1.010	0.048	0.048	1.696	1.461	0.039	0.022
Lab 9	36	1.667	0.954	0.050	0.049	1.683	1.541	0.074	0.035
Lab 10	34	1.599	0.937	0.021	0.021	1.703	1.514	0.046	0.022

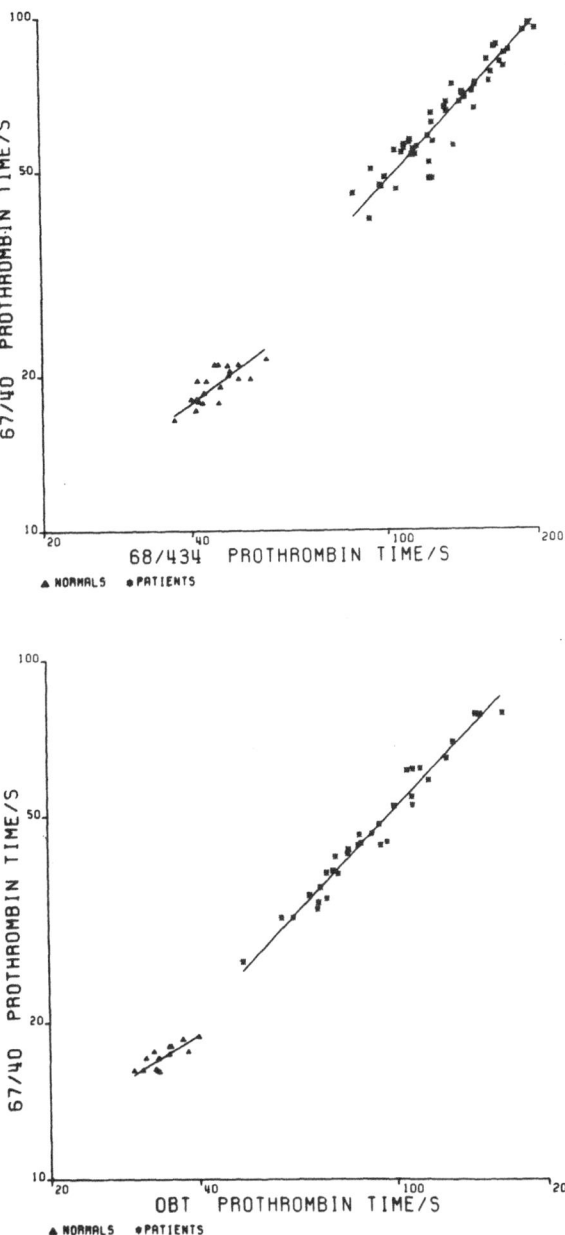

FIGURE 1: Two examples of data with orthogonal regression lines for the patients and for the normals non-coinciding.

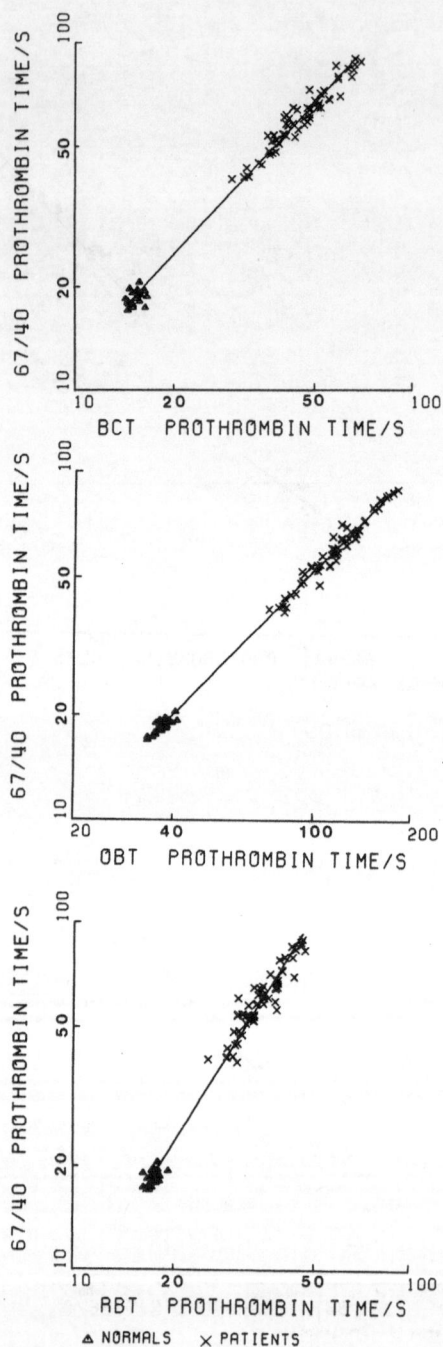

FIGURE 2: Three data sets with coinciding orthogonal regression lines for patients and for normals.

Fig. 2 gives an example of the data for one laboratory and three thromboplastins, with the orthogonal regression lines based on the combined data of patients and normals. Table 4 summarizes the results of the calculations for the five thromboplastins and the ten laboratories (European 1-7, American 8-10). The resulting calibration lines for each laboratory separately are shown in Fig. 3. Combination of the lines of the different laboratories to one final calibration line is done by taking the unweighted mean of the orthogonal regression lines, i.e., the mean of the slopes and the mean of the intercepts. As mentioned before, the final calibration lines will be based on the seven European laboratories who attended the workshop prior to the study. These results are given in Table 5.

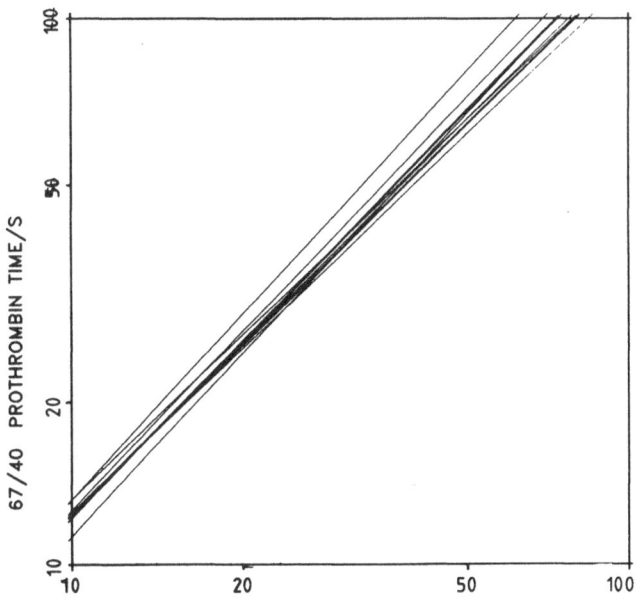

BCT PROTHROMBIN TIME/S

FIGURE 3A: The BCT/099 calibration lines for each of the ten laboratories. Each line is the orthogonal regression line relating the log seconds of the prothrombin times of the two thromboplastins (67/40 versus BCT/099).

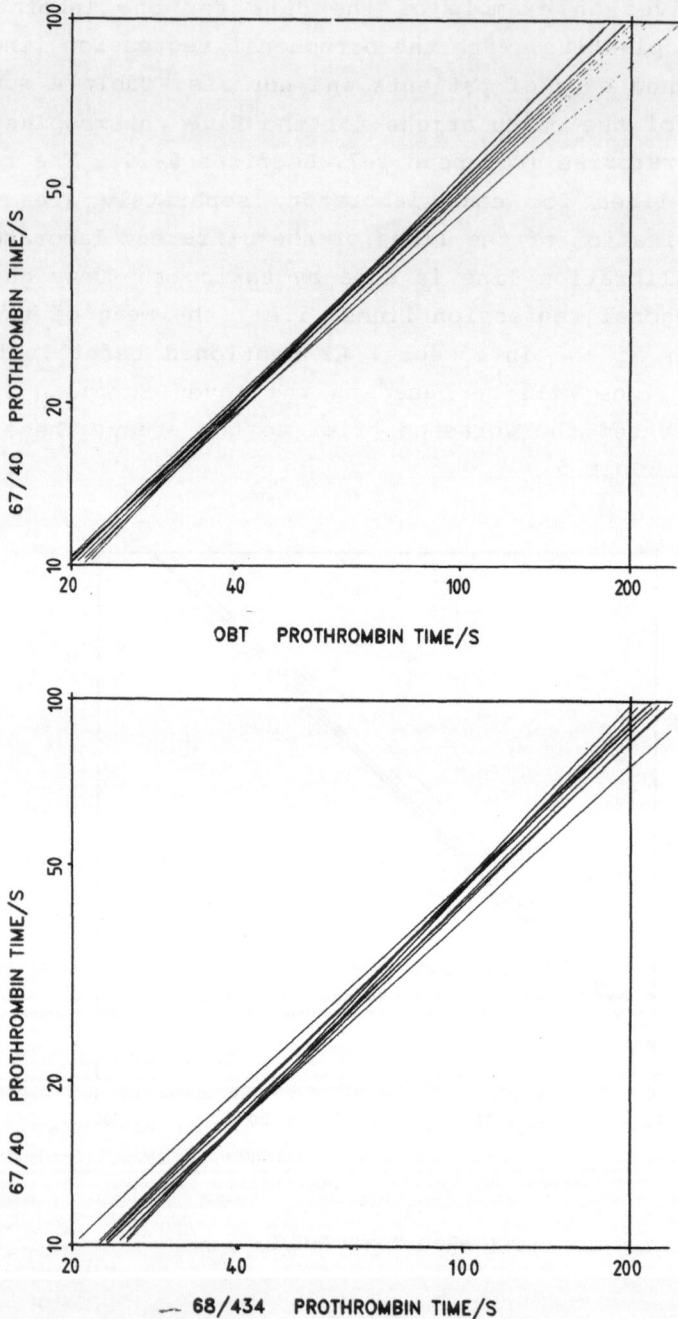

FIGURE 3B: The calibration lines of the two bovine tissue type thromboplastins for each of the ten laboratories (67/40 versus the secondary references OBT/79 and 68/434).

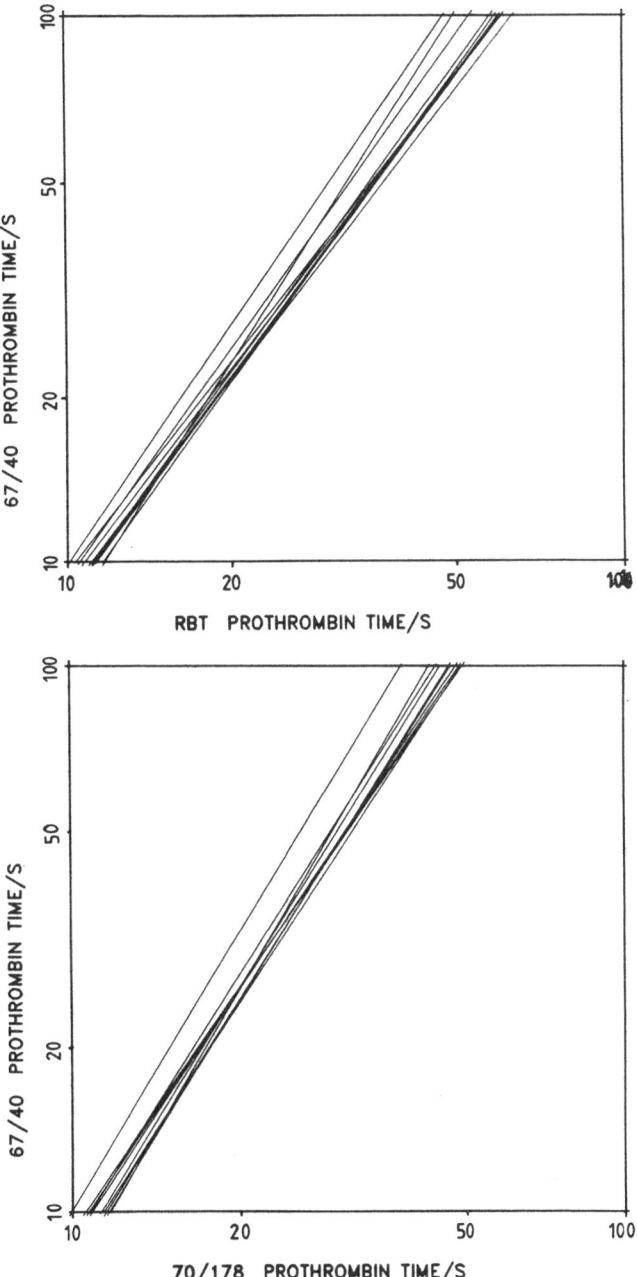

FIGURE 3C. The calibration lines of the two rabbit tissue type thromboplastins for each of the ten laboratories (67/40 versus the secondary references RBT/79 and 70/178).

Table 5 Unweighted means of the seven orthogonal regression lines y = a + bx for the five thromboplastins BCT/099, OBT/79, RBT/79, 68/434 and 70/178 (x-axis) versus 67/40 (y-axis). x and y are in log (time/s). Results of the seven European laboratories

	Inter-cept	Slope[1]	Between laboratories		Intercept in therapeutic range		Between labora-tories
	a	b	s_a	s_b	x	I	s_I
BCT/099	0.041	1.048	0.045	0.040	1.6	1.718	0.031
OBT/79	−0.321	1.011	0.065	0.040	2.0	1.701	0.018
RBT/79	−0.468	1.413	0.110	0.096	1.5	1.652	0.050
68/434	−0.410	1.027	0.074	0.042	2.0	1.645	0.015
70/178	−0.689	1.617	0.096	0.074	1.5	1.736	0.049

[1]) also called the international sensitivity index

3.2. Comparison with previous WHO calibration

For the present data we have also applied the original Biggs-Denson procedure. Table 6 summarizes the calibration constants calculated for each lab and each thromboplastin; moreover the WHO calibration constants are given, see (11) and (12).

Table 6 Calibration constants according to the Biggs Denson procedure

	68/434	70/178	BCT/099	OBT/79	RBT/79
Lab 1	0.94	0.46	0.83	0.98	0.54
Lab 2	1.04	0.58	0.97	1.08	0.68
Lab 3	0.97	0.42	0.89	1.00	0.48
Lab 4	1.00	0.50	0.85	0.99	0.61
Lab 5	0.98	0.47	0.98	0.95	0.62
Lab 6	0.85	0.46	0.99	0.89	0.58
Lab 7	0.85	0.51	0.90	0.89	0.58
Lab 8	0.99	0.54	1.03	0.97	0.65
Lab 9	0.93	0.53	0.81	0.91	0.59
Lab 10	1.11	0.53	1.00	1.18	0.58
Mean	0.966	0.500	0.925	0.984	0.591
s.d.	0.080	0.048	0.079	0.090	0.056
C.V. (%)	8.3	9.6	8.5	9.1	9.5
WHO	1.0	0.6			

4. DISCUSSION

In a collaborative study in accordance with a strict protocol five secondary reference thromboplastins were related to the primary international WHO reference preparation 67/40. No serious technical difficulties concerning the protocol were reported by the ten laboratories. The results show at several points differences between the laboratories, see e.g. the mean normal times (Table 5) and the calibration constants according to Biggs-Denson (Table 6). Drawing of conclusions from these differences is hampered by the fact that the laboratories did not test the same plasmas. The discrepancies, e.g. between the mean normal times, may be due to procedural differences or to properties of the population from which normals were taken.

Concerning the calibration constants in accordance with the Biggs-Denson procedure, we found for OBT/79 a range from 0.89 to 1.18 and for RBT/79 even from 0.48 to 0.68. For 68/434, the WHO previously established a constant of 1.0, whereas the present data give 0.966; similar figures for 70/178 are 0.6 and 0.500, respectively. The discrepancy for 70/178 might be related to a combination of a different level of anticoagulation and inadequacy of the Biggs-Denson procedure. Although in most cases the Biggs-Denson procedure fitted reasonably well to the data, some exceptions were found (see Fig. 4).

The alternative approach, i.e. relating log seconds obtained with one thromboplastin to those with another, did not show, at least with our data set, serious problems relating to this assumption. Differences between the laboratories are clearly present, see Fig. 3 and Table 4. An interesting point is how the three laboratories which did not attend the workshop to test the protocol, compare to the seven laboratories that did and which delivered the calibration line. To make such a comparison we have to compare the results of laboratories 8,9 and 10, given in Table 4, to the combined results of the seven laboratories in Table 5. A simple way to perform this comparison is to restrict our attention to slope b, and to calculate on the basis of Table 5 for each thromboplastin a 95% confidence interval for b taking into account the between-laboratory variability, i.e. $b \pm 2.45 s_b$,

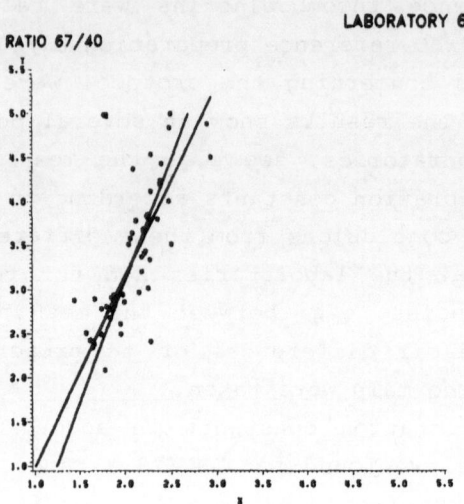

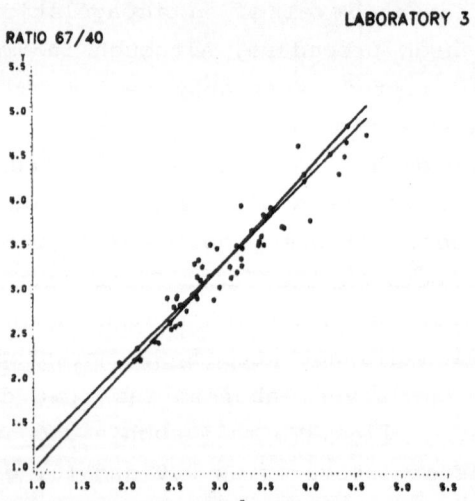

FIGURE 4: Two examples of ratio plots where the orthogonal regression line differs significantly from the Biggs Denson line, i.e., the line crossing (1,1) and the mean values.

and finally to check whether the slopes for labs 8, 9 and 10 lie within the interval. The 15 checks, which can be performed, led in one case (Lab 10, OBT/79) to a b value outside the confidence interval. This result is not alarming.

When establishing the calibration relation for a prothrombin time measured with a local thromboplastin, it should be recognized that a hierarchy of several calibration steps has been used. In general, the local thromboplastin is not directly calibrated against a WHO or BCR reference thromboplastin, but via one or more intermediate thromboplastins. A local batch should be related to a house standard; this house standard to the secondary reference material of its own tissue type; finally, the secondary reference material to the primary one. Figure 5 illustrates the hierarchy. The calibration relation studied here is only the final step in the hierarchy.

It should be kept in mind that the linearity of the relationship in log seconds for the combined patients' and normals' data

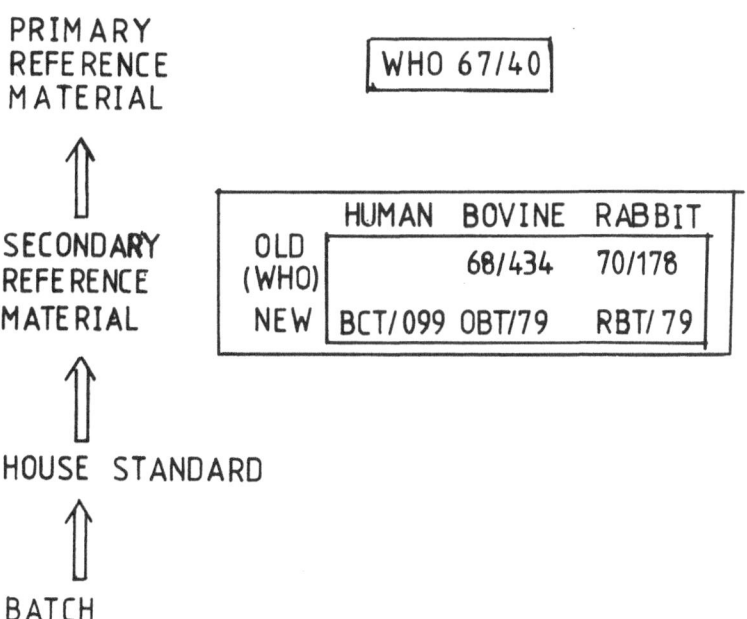

FIGURE 5: The hierarchy of several calibration steps.

is, just as for the Biggs-Denson relationship, empirically found and still has no theoretical foundation. For the five thromboplastins which we have studied in the final step of the hierarchy, the same linear relation for patients and normals fitted well. For other steps of the hierarchy this relation should, however, allways be checked very carefully. If a different linear relationship for patients and normals occurs, the transformation of ratios in accordance with equation 2 is not a priori justified. In some cases additional evidence might be available to justify ignoring the non-coincidence of the two lines. For example, in Fig. 1 the greater reliability of the patients' line and the fact that the patients' line crosses the normal scatter, was considered as such additional evidence.

5. ACKNOWLEDGEMENTS

The participating laboratories were:

Institut für Experimentelle Hämatologie und Bluttransfusionswesen der Universität Bonn, German Federal Republic (H. Beeser)

St. George's Hospital Medical School, London, Great Britain (P.T. Flute)

RELAC-Laboratorium, Academisch Ziekenhuis, Leiden, The Netherlands (E.A. Loeliger)

Københavns Amts Sygehus/Herlev, Herlev, Denmark (V.G. Nielsen)

Laboratoire Central d'Hématologie, Hôtel Dieu de Paris, Paris, France (M. Samama)

Istituto Superiore di Sanità, Roma, Italy (L. Tentori)

Afdeling Interne Geneeskunde, Universiteit Leuven, Leuven, Belgium (M. Verstraete and J. Vermylen)

CDC, Atlanta, Georgia, USA (B.L. Evatt)

NIH, Bethesda, Maryland, USA (H.R. Gralnick)

Ball Memorial Hospital, Muncie, Indiana, USA (D.A. Triplett).

The World Health Organization, Geneva, and the National Institute for Biological Standards and Control, London, are acknowledged for supplying the International Reference Preparations of Thromboplastin.

Very substantial contributions to the developed statistical calibration methodology were made by T.B.L. Kirkwood, National Institute for Biological Standards and Control, London, Great Britain and by M. Weis Bentzon, Statens Serum Institut, Copenhagen, Denmark.

REFERENCES

1. WHO Expert Committee on Biological Standardization. 28th Report. WHO Technical Report Series 610, World Health Organization, Geneva 1977: pp 14-15 and 45-51.
2. WHO Expert Committee on Biological Standardization. 31th Report. WHO Technical Report Series 658, World Health Organization, Geneva 1981: pp 185-205.
3. Biggs R, Denson KWE. Standardization of the one-stage prothrombin time for the control of anticoagulant therapy. Br Med J 1967; 1: 84-88.
4. Loeliger EA, Lewis SM. Progress in laboratory control of oral anticoagulants. Lancet 1982; II: 318-320.
5. Kirkwood TBL. Calibration of reference thromboplastins and standardisation of the prothrombin time ratio. Thromb Haemostas 1983; 49: 238-244.
6. Loeliger EA, Van den Besselaar AMHP, Hermans J, Van der Velde EA. Certification of three reference materials for thromboplastins. BCR information. Commission of the European Communities, Brussels, 1981.
7. WHO Expert Committee on Biological Standardization. 33rd Report. WHO Technical Report Series 687. World Health Organization, Geneva 1983: pp. 81-105.
8. Cornbleet PJ, Gochman N. Incorrect least-squares regression coefficients in method-comparison analysis. Clin Chem 1979; 25: 432-438.
9. Patefield WM. On the information matrix in the linear functional relationship problem. Appl Stat 1977; 26: 69-70.
10. Van der Velde EA. Orthogonal regression equation. This volume, chapter 3.
11. Bangham DR, Biggs R, Brozovic M, Denson KWE. Draft report of a collaborative study of two thromboplastins. In: Koller F, Brinkhous KM, Biggs R, Rodman NF, Hinnom S (eds.). Vascular Factors and Thrombosis. Schattauer, Stuttgart - New York 1970: pp 341-351.
12. Bangham DR, Biggs R, Brozovic M, Denson KWE. Calibration of five different thromboplastins, using fresh and freeze-dried plasma. Thrombos Diathes Haemorrh 1973; 29: 228-239.

ANNEX 1: ANALYTICAL PROTOCOL FOR THE CHARACTERIZATION OF THE BCR
REFERENCE MATERIALS FOR THROMBOPLASTINS (with 5 appendices)

1. INTRODUCTION

The present protocol was designed to obtain certified reference materials (RMs) for thromboplastins used in oral anticoagulant control in the European Economic Communities. It is the
result of the cooperative effort of a group of experts of the
seven countries belonging to the European Economic Communities,
and was prepared according to recommendations of the International Committee for Standardization in Haematology. The document
also satisfies the Proposed Requirements laid down by WHO. To
make the results of the study useful also for possible future
replacement of the present WHO reference thromboplastins, 3
American laboratories were asked to take part in the study. The
total of laboratories participating in the study shall be 10, 7
European and 3 American (see APPENDIX 5, pp. 75-76).

2. EXPERIMENTAL DESIGN

Testing of thromboplastins by the 10 participating laboratories should be completed within 5 weeks after receipt of the
material. All laboratories shall test the thromboplastins on at
least 6 days (with an optional maximum of 10 days), using on each
day freshly prepared plasmas of 2 normal individuals and 6
patients. A one-day experiment should be completed 5 hours after
the start of the collection of blood. The schedule of a one-day
experiment is as follows :

2.1. First 1-2 hours: Collection of blood and preparation of
thromboplastin suspension. The blood will be drawn from 2 normal
subjects (see 3.1.) and 6 patients stabilized on oral anticoagulation (see 3.2.). To separate plasma from red cells,

centrifugation will take place immediately after withdrawal of the blood, after which the plasma will be transferred to another tube. The latter tube will be stoppered and held at room temperature until used for testing.

2.2. Second part (2-3 hours): Actual testing of the 8 plasma samples with 6 thromboplastins according to the statistical design, presented in APPENDIX 3 (p. 72). Instructions to be consulted immediately before testing are given in APPENDIX 2 (p. 71), and APPENDIX 4 (pp. 73-74) is an example of a data sheet to be used in actual testing.

Note 1: Testing shall not be done in duplicate but in single determinations.

The main reason for using duplicate determinations would be (a) outlier detection and (b) estimation of residual errors. However, in this study the detection of serious outliers will be facilitated by the multiple testing of each individual plasma using 6 thromboplastins. Furthermore, the variation between duplicates will make only a relatively small contribution to the total variability in the data.

Single determinations are also preferable to duplicate determinations, because it is important to minimize the total duration of the testing procedure in order to avoid serious bias due to time effects.

Note 2: The 6 determinations (one with each thromboplastin) for each subject (normal or patient) shall be performed immediately after each other. Thus, all determinations of the previous subject should be completed before starting a new series of 6 determinations with the next subject's plasma.

This order of testing means that determinations for each subject will be tied together as closely as possible in time. This should minimize the effect of temporal drift on the comparison between thromboplastins.

Note 3: The order in which the patients are tested shall be random. To achieve this, the order of testing of patient samples should be the same as the order of collection if the latter is considered to be random. In any case, the order of testing should <u>not</u> be related to the prolongation of the clotting time in the patient. The collection of normal 1 (which will be tested first) shall be before patient sample collection, while the collection of normal 2 (which will be tested last) shall be after patient sample collection.

3. SELECTION OF NORMALS AND PATIENTS

3.1. <u>Normals</u>

The <u>normal</u> subjects must be ambulant adults (females may be included irrespective of whether they are taking oral contraceptives). If possible, for a one-day experiment, use one male and one female. <u>Take a different pair of normals each day</u>.

3.2. <u>Patients</u>

Take <u>patients</u> who have recovered their general health (hence preferably out-patients) and who have been <u>stabilized on anticoagulants for at least 6 weeks</u>. <u>All levels of intensity of treatment are acceptable provided the patients display stable anticoagulation</u>.

Laboratories with access to a large number of patients are requested to select the 6 patient samples displaying the widest possible variety of levels of anticoagulation. This means, in terms of British Ratio, from 1.5 to 5 times prolongation of the prothrombin time.

Laboratories having only few patients should take 6 samples irrespective of their level of anticoagulation. <u>Take each day a different set of 6 patients</u>.

To avoid unwanted bias, <u>all results obtained with samples once chosen for investigation must be reported</u>.

4. SAMPLE COLLECTION

4.1. Nine volumes of blood shall be collected by clean venepuncture, into one volume of <u>sterile trisodium citrate 0.109 M (provided)</u>; blood should be drawn <u>either</u> with a plastic syringe and transferred into a plastic tube <u>or</u> with other non-contact-activation equipment.

4.2. The blood shall be <u>centrifuged</u> immediately after collection, with an ordinary bench-centrifuge (appr. 800 g = 2,500 rpm), for <u>5 minutes</u>, at room temperature.

4.3. The plasma shall be <u>transferred</u> by means of a non-contact pipette to a stoppered non-contact tube, and then <u>stoppered</u>.

4.4. The stoppered test tube containing plasma is kept at <u>room temperature</u> until testing.

5. HANDLING OF THROMBOPLASTINS

Six different thromboplastin preparations will be tested. Three of the 6 are the current WHO reference thromboplastins which are under the custodianship of the National Institute for Biological Standards and Control in London. The preparations are: human brain, <u>combined</u>, thromboplastin 67/40; bovine brain, <u>combined</u>, thromboplastin 68/434; and rabbit brain, <u>plain</u>, thromboplastin 70/178. The other 3 thromboplastins are: human brain, <u>plain</u>, a batch of British Comparative Thromboplastin (BCT/099); bovine brain, <u>combined</u> (called here OBT/79); and rabbit brain, <u>plain</u> (called here RBT/79).

Note: Thromboplastin <u>combined</u> means: containing fibrinogen, factor V and calcium (the latter after reconstitution). Thromboplastin <u>plain</u> means: not containing fibrinogen and factor V.

Upon receipt, the thromboplastins shall be <u>stored</u> refrigerated (<u>4-10°C</u>).

<u>Preparation for use of thromboplastins</u>

a. Thromboplastin 67/40: reconstitute 2 ampoules with 2.0 ml of 3.2 mM $CaCl_2$ (<u>provided</u>) each. Please pool.
   The normal prothrombin time obtained with thromboplastin 67/40 is 19 sec ± 2 sec (SD).
   Keep at room temperature until use.

b. Thromboplastin 68/434: reconstitute 2 ampoules with 2.2 ml of 3.2 mM $CaCl_2$ (<u>provided</u>) each. Please pool.
   The normal prothrombin time obtained with this thromboplastin is approximately 40 sec (range 34-52).
   Keep at room temperature until use.

c. Thromboplastin 70/178: reconstitute 1 ampoule with 1.0 ml distilled water (provided). Leave thromboplastin in the ampoule.

The normal prothrombin time obtained with this preparation is approximately 17 sec.

Note: this thromboplastin does not contain calcium.

Keep at room temperature until use.

d. Thromboplastin BCT/099 (human brain, plain): reconstitute 1 vial with 1.0 ml phenolized water (provided). Leave thromboplastin in the vial.

The normal prothrombin time obtained with BCT is approximately 13.5 sec.

Note: this thromboplastin does not contain calcium.

Keep at room temperature until use.

e. Thromboplastin OBT/79 (bovine brain, combined): reconstitute 2 ampoules with 2.2 ml of 3.2 mM $CaCl_2$ (provided) each. Please pool.

The normal prothrombin times with this thromboplastin display a range similar to that found for thromboplastin 68/434.

Keep at room temperature until use.

f. Thromboplastin RBT/79 (rabbit brain, plain): reconstitute 3 ampoules with 0.5 ml (not 1.0 ml as for 70/178) distilled water (provided) each; please pool.

The normal prothrombin time with this thromboplastin is in the same range as for thromboplastin 70/178.

Note: This thromboplastin does not contain calcium.

Keep at room temperature until use.

6. OTHER REAGENTS (provided)

sterile sodium citrate 0.109 M	: for blood collection;
sterile water	: for reconstitution of thromboplastin 70/178 and RBT/79;
phenolized water (0.05%)	: for reconstitution of thromboplastin BCT/099;

sterile CaCl$_2$ 3.2 mM	: for reconstitution of thromboplastin 67/40, 68/434 and OBT/79;
sterile CaCl$_2$ 25 mM	: for recalcification of plasma/thromboplastin mixture (thromboplastin 70/178, BCT/099 and RBT/79).

7. EQUIPMENT (please fill in APPENDIX 1, p. 70)

Non-contact syringes and/or test tubes for blood collection.

Non-contact test tubes with non-contact stopper (do not use rubber stoppers!) for storage of blood or plasma.

Non-contact pipettes for transfer of plasma from (centrifuged) blood tubes into tubes for storage of plasma.

Non-contact pipettes for transfer of plasma into glass test tubes at the time of testing.

Usual glass test tubes for the actual testing (glass tubes shall be provided to the American laboratories, if needed).

Thermostat ("water-bath") with water temperature of 37°C (tolerance limits: 37.0±0.2). Use calibrated thermometer!

8. ACTUAL TESTING (before doing so, consult APPENDIX 2, p. 71 containing "Instructions for actual testing").

All participants use their own pipettes, test tubes, dispensers and thermostats. Fresh pipetting tips shall be used for each test.

To facilitate the determinations, the sequence of testing per sample is arranged such that the 3 thromboplastins with an amount of 0.4 ml and those with an amount of 0.1 ml are consecutive (see APPENDIX 3, p. 72).

The actual testing shall be performed on each day as follows:

first series:

normal 1 shall be tested with all 6 thromboplastin in the order indicated on the data sheet (Note: each day there is another order of thromboplastins).

second series:

next, patient 1 shall be tested with all 6 thromboplastins in the same order.

third series:

next, patient 2 ditto.

fourth series:

next, patient 3 ditto.

fifth series:

next, patient 4 ditto.

sixth series:

next, patient 5 ditto.

seventh series:

next, patient 6 ditto.

eighth series:

next, normal 2 ditto.

The coagulation endpoint shall be determined by hand and eye, preferably with the so-called tilt-tube technique (coagulation endpoints obtained with thromboplastin 68/434 and OBT have to be determined with the tilt-tube technique, the Kolle-hook reading being inaccurate. The Kolle-hook technique might be used for reading endpoints obtained with 67/40, 70/178, BCT and RBT. If the tilt-tube technique is used, test tubes must be kept as deep as possible under water in order to maintain optimal temperature (50 mm appears to be optimal as stated by Uldall; but 30 mm should do equally well for participants using small test tubes). The use of an illuminated water-bath minimizes the necessity for removal of the tube from the water!

For each of the eight series the following procedure shall be applied for the 6 determinations with the 6 different thromboplastins:

1. Place 6 ordinary glass tubes in the water-bath (plastic tubes may be used).

2. Transfer the correct amount of thromboplastin in each of the 6 tubes. The appropriate amounts are 0.4 ml for thromboplastin 67/40, 68/434 and OBT/79; 0.1 ml for 70/178, BCT/099 and RBT/79. The order in which these thromboplastins are used is different for each day and is indicated on the data sheet.

3. If the tube contains 0.4 ml thromboplastin with calcium (67/40, 68/434 and OBT/79), the next steps are as follows:
   a. make sure that <u>2 min</u> have passed between transferral of the thromboplastin into tube 1 and further processing (for plastic tubes the warming up time will be 3-4 min);
   b. transfer 0.05 ml <u>not</u> prewarmed plasma to the test tube;
   c. start the stopwatch immediately and mix;
   d. read the coagulation endpoint.

or 4. If the tube contains <u>0.1 ml</u> thromboplastin without calcium (70/178, BCT/099 and RBT/79):
   a. ensure that 2 min have passed between transferral of the thromboplastin into tube 1 and further processing (for plastic tubes warming up will take 3-4 min);
   b. add 0.1 ml not prewarmed plasma to the test tube;
   c. mix thoroughly with the thromboplastin;
   d. wait 1 min for incubation to reach the optimal reaction temperature (in plastic tubes 3 min);
   e. recalcify with 0.1 ml prewarmed $CaCl_2$ (25 mM) <u>after</u> the end of this 1 min incubation period;
   f. read the clotting endpoint with the hand-reading technique as customary in your laboratory (see previous page).

Because of the 3-minute incubation time needed to prewarm the various reaction mixtures (2 min* for the first tube of each series to prewarm thromboplastin, and 3 times 1 min* for pre-warming the plasma thromboplastin mixture in tubes containing thromboplastin plain), and because of the long prothrombin times expected with thromboplastins 68/434 and OBT/79 (for patient samples up to more than 3 min), one series will take 12-18 min, and the testing of 8 samples about 2 hours (if plastic tubes are used for testing, considerably more time is required).

---

*with plastic tubes: 3-4 min.

9. AMOUNT OF REAGENTS AND AMPOULES NEEDED PER DAY

Thromboplastins

Thromboplastins combined (67/40, 68/434 and OBT/79): 2 ampoules; thromboplastins plain (70/178): 1 ampoule; BCT/099: 1 vial; RBT/79: 3 ampoules.

Other reagents

Citrate, water, phenolized water, $CaCl_2$ 3.2 mM, $CaCl_2$ 25 mM - fresh vials each day.

Plasma

Approximately 0.5 ml (3 times 0.05 ml for thromboplastins combined, and 3 times 0.1 ml for thromboplastins plain; together amounting to 0.45 ml). To provide for unforeseen circumstances, a minimum of 0.5 ml per sample should be available.

10. MAILING OF DATA SHEETS (minimal 6)

Please keep the original set of forms for your files. Send 1 photocopy to:

> Dr. E.A. van der Velde
> Department of Medical Statistics
> University of Leiden
> Wassenaarseweg 80, P.O. Box 9512
> 2300 RA LEIDEN, The Netherlands
> Tel.: 71 (Leiden) 148333, ext. 5150/5009/5148

and a second photocopy to:

> Prof. M. Hjelm
> Community Bureau of Reference (BCR)
> 8, Square de Méeûs
> B-1049 BRUSSELS, Belgium

The filled-in APPENDIX 1 should also be sent to Dr. E.A. van der Velde, Leiden, and to Prof. M. Hjelm, BCR, Brussels.

LITERATURE

1. Biggs R, Denson KWE. Standardization of the one-stage prothrombin time for the control of anticoagulant therapy. Br Med J 1967; 1: 84.

2. Denson KWE. International and national standardization of the control of anticoagulant therapy in patients receiving coumarin and indanedione drugs using calibrated thromboplastin preparations. J Clin Pathol 1971; 24: 460.
3. Ingram GIC, Hills M. The prothrombin time test: effect of varying citrate concentration. Thromb Haemostas 1976; 36: 230.
4. Ingram GIC, Hills M. Reference method for the one-stage prothrombin time test on human blood. Thromb Haemostas 1976; 36: 237.
5. Uldall A. Prothrombin time standardization and temperature problems. Clin Chim Acta 1980; 103: 39-44.
6. WHO Expert Committee on Biological Standardization. 28th Report. WHO Technical Report Series 610, World Health Organization, Geneva 1977: pp. 45-51.

APPENDIX 1 Medical and Technical Information
LABORATORY ...

A. ANTICOAGULANTS USED FOR PATIENT TREATMENT

☐ Acenocoumarol
☐ Dicoumarol
☐ Phenindion
☐ Phenprocoumon
☐ Warfarin
☐ other (specify: ....).

B. ANTICOAGULANT FOR DECALCIFICATION OF PATIENT'S BLOOD

☐ 0.11 M citrate (3.2%)
☐ 0.13 M citrate (3.8%)
☐ other (specify: ....)

C. BUFFERING OF CITRATE

☐ no
☐ with HEPES 66 g/l
☐ citric acid (specify: ....)
☐ other (specify: ....)

only to be filled in if, in case of lack of provided material local reagent is used

D. EQUIPMENT FOR BLOOD COLLECTION

☐ siliconized syringe
☐ plastic syringe (manuf.: ....)

Composition: if siliconized syringes are used, siliconized by:
  ☐ manufacturer
  ☐ laboratory

E. CONTAINER FOR BLOOD STORAGE

☐ siliconized glass tubes
☐ plastic tubes (manuf.: ....)

if siliconized tubes are used, siliconization by
  ☐ manufacturer
  ☐ laboratory

F. SIZE OF TUBES FOR ACTUAL TESTING

Diameter: .... mm
Height : .... mm

G. MATERIAL OF TUBES FOR ACTUAL TESTING

☐ glass
☐ plastic

H. COAGULATION ENDPOINT READING

☐ tilt-tube (if yes, for which thromboplastins:
  ....)
☐ loop or Kolle-hook (if yes, for which thromboplastins:
  ....)

APPENDIX 2 Instructions for Actual Testing

1. Make sure each day that you are using the appropriate DATA SHEET, and that you have sorted out the 6 thromboplastins in the correct order indicated on the SHEET.

2. Before you start, please check the following experimental details:

   a) correct volumes of the pipettes to be used;
   b) correct reconstituents for thromboplastins (type and amount);
   c) correct order of thromboplastins;
   d) clean test tubes;
   e) stop watch warmed up;
   f) waterbath 37°C
   g) mix-o-matic working

3. Examples of how to fill in the observed prothrombin times: for 138.4 seconds and 87.3 seconds, write:

   | 1 | 3 | 8 | . | 4 |
   | | 8 | 7 | . | 3 |

4. You should record all data, including those you consider incorrect. In that case, indicate the reason(s) under COMMENTS.

   Example:

   Patient 1

   11 | 8 | 2 | 7 | . | 4 |

   Patient 2

   28 | 0 | 0 | 5 | . | 2 |

   COMMENTS: 11 Wrong type of reagents
            28 Wrong sequence of reagents

5. If a determination has not been performed for some reason, do not fill in the corresponding boxes.

APPENDIX 3

The order of thromboplastins on the consecutive days has to be as follows:

Order of thrombo-plastins	Number of days						Optional		
	1	2	3	4	5	6	7	8	9
1	BCT	67/40	OBT	RBT	68/434	70/178	67/40	BCT	OBT
2	70/178	OBT	67/40	BCT	67/40	BCT	OBT	RBT	68/434
3	RBT	68/434	68/434	70/178	OBT	RBT	68/434	70/178	67/40
4	68/434	70/178	RBT	67/40	BCT	OBT	70/178	OBT	BCT
5	OBT	RBT	70/178	68/434	RBT	68/434	RBT	67/40	70/178
6	67/40	BCT	BCT	OBT	70/178	67/40	BCT	68/434	RBT

order given in Example of Data Sheet (APPENDIX 4, pp. 73-74)

where:

	old	new
human	67/40	BCT
bovine	68/434	OBT
rabbit	70/178	RBT

N.B.: BCT = BCT/099
OBT = OBT/79
RBT = RBT/79

APPENDIX 4 Example of Data Sheet for the Characterization of the BCR Reference Materials for Thromboplastins (Note: each sheet displays another order of thromboplastins).

DAY 3

Start of collection	.... hrs .... min
Start of determination	.... hrs .... min
End of determination	.... hrs .... min
Room temperature at the start of collection	...... °C
Room temperature at the end of determination	...... °C
Water-bath temperature	...... °C

Laboratory/Punch card number ☐☐ ☐ 1

month   day

Date of testing (April 3 = 0 4 0 3) ☐☐ ☐☐

PROTHROMBIN TIME IN SECONDS:

Order of thrombo-plastins*	Tube	Series 1 (Normal 1)	Tube	Series 2 (Patient 1)	Tube	Series 3 (Patient 2)
OBT	1	☐☐☐ . ☐	7	☐☐☐ . ☐	13	☐☐☐ . ☐
67/40	2	☐☐☐ . ☐	8	☐☐☐ . ☐	14	☐☐☐ . ☐
68/434	3	☐☐☐ . ☐	9	☐☐☐ . ☐	15	☐☐☐ . ☐
RBT	4	☐☐☐ . ☐	10	☐☐☐ . ☐	16	☐☐☐ . ☐
70/178	5	☐☐☐ . ☐	11	☐☐☐ . ☐	17	☐☐☐ . ☐
BCT	6	☐☐☐ . ☐	12	☐☐☐ . ☐	18	☐☐☐ . ☐

COMMENTS (for the whole series of determinations (2 normals + 6 patients)):

*Note: order is different for each day (see APPENDIX 3, p. 72).

DAY 3

Laboratory/Punch card number   ☐☐ 2

Date of testing (April 3 = 0 4   0 3)   month ☐☐   day ☐☐

PROTHROMBIN TIME IN SECONDS:

Order of thrombo-plastins*	Tube	Series 4 (Patient 3)	Tube	Series 5 (Patient 4)	Tube	Series 6 (Patient 5)
OBT	19	☐☐☐ · ☐	25	☐☐☐ · ☐	31	☐☐☐ · ☐
67/40	20	☐☐☐ · ☐	26	☐☐☐ · ☐	32	☐☐☐ · ☐
68/434	21	☐☐☐ · ☐	27	☐☐☐ · ☐	33	☐☐☐ · ☐
RBT	22	☐☐☐ · ☐	28	☐☐☐ · ☐	34	☐☐☐ · ☐
70/178	23	☐☐☐ · ☐	29	☐☐☐ · ☐	35	☐☐☐ · ☐
BCT	24	☐☐☐ · ☐	30	☐☐☐ · ☐	36	☐☐☐ · ☐

Laboratory/Punch card number   ☐☐ 3

Date of testing (April 3 = 0 4   0 3)   month ☐☐   day ☐☐

PROTHROMBIN TIME IN SECONDS:

Order of thrombo-plastins*	Tube	Series 7 (Patient 6)	Tube	Series 8 (Normal 2)	
OBT	37	☐☐☐ · ☐	43	☐☐☐ · ☐	sex of the two
67/40	38	☐☐☐ · ☐	44	☐☐☐ · ☐ ,	normals:
68/434	39	☐☐☐ · ☐	45	☐☐☐ · ☐	Male = 1
RBT	40	☐☐☐ · ☐	46	☐☐☐ · ☐	Female = 2
70/178	41	☐☐☐ · ☐	47	☐☐☐ · ☐	1st normal ☐
BCT	42	☐☐☐ · ☐	48	☐☐☐ · ☐	2nd normal ☐

*Please note change in order for consecutive days (see APPENDIX 3, p. 72).

APPENDIX 5

European laboratories:

Dr. H. Beeser and Miss H. Nass
Institut für experimentelle Hämatologie
Universität Bonn
53 BONN VENUSBERG
Annabergerweg
Germany

Prof. P.T. Flute and Miss V. Muffty
St. George's Hospital
Medical School
Cranmer Terrace
LONDON SW17 0RE
Great Britain

Prof.dr. E.A. Loeliger and Mrs. L.P. van Halem
Academisch Ziekenhuis
Afdeling Interne Geneeskunde
Rijnsburgerweg 10
2333 AA LEIDEN
The Netherlands

Dr. V.G. Nielsen and Mr. A. Uldall
Herlev Hospital
University of Copenhagen
Ringvejen
DK 2730 HERLEV
Denmark

Prof. M. Samama and Mrs. S. Ionescu
Laboratoire Central d'Hématologie
Hôtel Dieu de Paris
1, Place du Parvis Notre Dame
75181 PARIS CEDEX 04
France

Prof. L. Tentori and Miss M. Orlando
Istituto Superiore di Sanità
Viale Regina Elena, 299
00161 ROMA
Italy

Prof. M. Verstraete and Mrs. L. Daniels
Universiteit Leuven
Afdeling Interne Geneeskunde
Kapucijnenvoer 35
3000 LEUVEN
Belgium

American laboratories

Dr. B.L. Evatt
Director Hematology
Department of Health, Education, and Welfare
Center for Disease Control
ATLANTA, Georgia 30333
U.S.A.

Dr. H.R. Gralnick
Hematology Service
Clinical Pathology Department
Clinical Center, Bldg. 10
Room 5N-236
National Institutes of Health
BETHESDA, Maryland 20014
U.S.A

Dr. D.A .Triplett
Ball Memorial Hospital
Department of Pathology
MUNCIE, Indiana 47303
U.S.A.

ANNEX 2: RAW DATA OF THE BCR THROMBOPLASTIN CALIBRATION STUDY

The first four columns represent respectively:
- laboratory code;
- day number;
- patient (P) or normal (N);
- sequence number within one day for patients and normals, respectively.

The last 6 columns represent the prothrombin times (in seconds x 10) for respectively:
- 67/40
- 68/434
- 70/178

- BCT/099
- OBT/79
- RBT/79

(0 is missing value).

1	1	P	1	54.0	129.8	27.2	34.5	113.1	36.2
1	1	P	2	48.2	106.8	25.2	30.8	100.4	31.5
1	1	P	3	38.8	86.5	21.4	23.3	80.0	24.4
1	1	P	4	32.6	80.4	21.2	24.8	71.0	24.8
1	1	P	5	36.5	93.0	22.7	25.7	85.9	26.4
1	1	P	6	65.0	128.7	27.8	38.7	126.2	31.4
1	2	P	1	44.9	113.0	27.2	34.0	106.1	31.2
1	2	P	2	52.6	125.4	27.3	34.0	114.0	34.0
1	2	P	3	52.0	113.7	28.0	35.0	104.3	30.2
1	2	P	4	46.6	116.2	26.0	32.7	108.9	28.3
1	2	P	5	61.2	130.6	29.0	41.0	134.2	34.0
1	2	P	6	60.8	146.6	33.5	45.8	139.8	39.0
1	3	P	1	49.7	103.2	24.1	30.1	95.5	27.0
1	3	P	2	49.9	107.5	25.7	31.1	98.6	28.8
1	3	P	3	49.2	126.4	25.0	33.1	111.7	28.0
1	3	P	4	46.8	116.0	24.4	31.1	103.2	28.2
1	3	P	5	47.5	112.2	23.7	30.6	105.2	26.8
1	3	P	6	45.7	131.0	24.3	31.8	109.8	26.0
1	4	P	1	62.4	130.1	29.9	38.8	129.6	34.4
1	4	P	2	50.2	113.4	24.4	30.4	101.4	26.0
1	4	P	3	31.7	70.7	19.6	21.7	65.2	21.1
1	4	P	4	43.6	93.2	25.0	30.6	82.2	27.5
1	4	P	5	50.7	117.2	28.4	36.2	112.5	33.5
1	4	P	6	63.0	146.0	32.9	40.1	134.7	38.8
1	5	P	1	39.2	82.0	20.3	23.9	74.3	26.1
1	5	P	2	32.3	80.6	20.0	23.2	71.0	22.8
1	5	P	3	50.3	113.6	25.2	32.8	102.4	31.0
1	5	P	4	35.1	67.8	21.9	22.5	62.5	22.9
1	5	P	5	45.1	113.8	24.7	30.2	104.2	28.8
1	5	P	6	38.6	98.5	22.1	23.8	81.5	24.6
1	6	P	1	45.8	106.7	25.0	30.6	98.6	28.8
1	6	P	2	30.0	65.1	19.0	22.4	61.6	21.1
1	6	P	3	61.2	143.0	29.0	42.8	134.8	35.3
1	6	P	4	42.7	91.6	23.0	28.1	87.0	25.6
1	6	P	5	96.5	216.2	38.8	65.5	196.9	51.0
1	6	P	6	43.4	99.0	22.6	28.3	90.0	25.2
1	7	P	1	39.9	104.0	22.7	27.8	90.5	25.2
1	7	P	2	104.8	287.7	41.0	61.6	298.8	52.2
1	7	P	3	52.5	102.0	26.0	34.0	98.1	30.2
1	7	P	4	73.1	189.0	34.8	52.5	180.0	40.7
1	7	P	5	45.3	100.0	24.6	29.0	94.9	27.6
1	7	P	6	29.9	74.5	20.7	20.2	62.0	23.0
1	8	P	1	67.2	154.2	33.6	44.8	155.0	41.5
1	8	P	2	36.4	84.0	22.6	24.1	76.5	23.0
1	8	P	3	41.2	102.0	23.7	26.8	90.2	23.6
1	8	P	4	45.5	102.7	26.4	30.5	100.8	26.1
1	8	P	5	24.4	54.0	16.5	16.8	48.5	17.0
1	8	P	6	61.7	167.2	27.7	37.5	135.7	30.2
1	9	P	1	59.8	131.3	30.0	40.2	227.2	33.6
1	9	P	2	75.0	170.4	34.5	59.6	163.6	40.0
1	9	P	3	55.4	116.5	26.7	37.9	107.2	28.8
1	9	P	4	55.2	130.6	27.1	39.7	112.0	30.7
1	9	P	5	57.2	121.0	27.4	36.4	105.0	29.3
1	9	P	6	39.2	89.8	22.4	27.1	79.4	23.2
1	10	P	1	43.3	102.6	21.7	27.3	88.8	25.9
1	10	P	2	47.9	106.2	23.8	32.0	94.9	28.8
1	10	P	3	87.0	218.8	41.9	64.7	207.4	58.2
1	10	P	4	44.7	105.7	25.0	32.5	96.4	28.8
1	10	P	5	64.0	132.5	30.5	50.7	128.5	35.4
1	10	P	6	46.8	109.7	24.4	30.3	102.7	28.5
1	1	N	1	17.2	44.0	14.8	13.2	38.0	15.0
1	1	N	2	16.4	37.0	13.2	12.4	35.2	14.1
1	2	N	1	16.4	41.6	13.7	12.2	36.8	14.2
1	2	N	2	15.8	37.4	13.4	12.6	34.6	14.0
1	3	N	1	17.3	44.5	14.5	14.0	38.0	15.5
1	3	N	2	18.0	45.0	14.8	14.5	39.0	15.5
1	4	N	1	16.5	39.3	13.8	12.8	34.0	15.4
1	4	N	2	16.6	39.4	14.0	12.2	33.8	15.5
1	5	N	1	16.3	39.0	13.7	12.8	32.4	14.6
1	5	N	2	16.5	38.1	13.5	13.0	33.0	15.0
1	6	N	1	17.0	41.9	14.6	14.0	38.4	15.7
1	6	N	2	18.0	42.0	13.1	13.0	35.9	14.3
1	7	N	1	17.7	41.2	14.2	13.0	35.8	14.8
1	7	N	2	17.8	39.2	14.0	13.2	35.3	14.9
1	8	N	1	19.8	55.3	14.9	14.4	48.2	15.9
1	8	N	2	16.0	35.5	12.5	11.3	31.6	12.8
1	9	N	1	18.0	40.8	14.0	13.0	36.0	14.4
1	9	N	2	17.2	41.2	13.7	12.7	35.6	14.3
1	10	N	1	17.0	37.3	12.4	12.5	33.6	12.5
1	10	N	2	17.0	39.3	13.6	12.9	35.2	14.2

2	1	P	1	37.0	79.0	22.0	27.0	72.0	25.0
2	1	P	2	39.5	93.0	28.5	36.5	83.0	35.0
2	1	P	3	36.0	83.0	23.0	29.0	71.0	27.0
2	1	P	4	51.0	123.0	30.0	42.0	102.5	36.5
2	1	P	5	42.0	83.0	26.0	37.5	76.0	33.0
2	1	P	6	32.5	80.0	24.0	29.5	70.0	28.0
2	2	P	1	33.5	80.0	23.5	27.5	72.0	26.5
2	2	P	2	39.5	103.5	27.0	34.5	91.5	31.5
2	2	P	3	43.5	105.0	30.0	35.0	95.5	36.5
2	2	P	4	34.5	72.5	24.0	30.0	65.0	29.5
2	2	P	5	46.0	106.0	28.5	38.0	94.5	35.0
2	2	P	6	35.0	90.0	25.0	31.0	76.5	31.5
2	3	P	1	23.0	55.5	19.0	17.5	48.5	20.5
2	3	P	2	31.0	79.5	25.5	26.0	69.5	29.0
2	3	P	3	39.0	96.0	26.5	32.0	82.0	31.5
2	3	P	4	27.5	68.0	21.5	21.0	59.5	24.0
2	3	P	5	54.0	115.5	30.0	40.5	100.0	38.0
2	3	P	6	49.5	94.0	28.0	33.5	83.0	33.0
2	4	P	1	36.5	88.5	28.0	28.5	77.0	34.0
2	4	P	2	41.0	90.5	26.5	30.0	82.0	32.0
2	4	P	3	25.0	60.5	20.0	18.5	50.5	23.0
2	4	P	4	35.0	88.5	26.0	27.5	75.0	30.5
2	4	P	5	37.5	86.0	28.0	31.0	76.5	34.0
2	4	P	6	44.0	115.0	32.5	35.5	98.0	38.5
2	5	P	1	34.5	80.5	25.0	27.0	70.0	29.5
2	5	P	2	39.5	106.0	29.0	32.0	90.0	35.0
2	5	P	3	24.5	52.5	17.5	18.0	45.5	20.0
2	5	P	4	37.0	77.0	26.0	28.5	68.0	30.0
2	5	P	5	46.0	99.5	28.0	34.0	88.5	34.0
2	5	P	6	23.0	56.5	18.5	18.0	49.0	20.5
2	6	P	1	47.0	118.0	29.0	41.0	101.0	35.0
2	6	P	2	33.0	80.5	26.0	27.0	71.5	29.5
2	6	P	3	50.0	125.5	31.5	40.0	107.5	38.0
2	6	P	4	50.5	124.5	34.0	44.0	107.0	42.0
2	6	P	5	52.5	111.5	33.5	42.0	103.0	41.0
2	6	P	6	30.5	70.5	24.0	24.0	62.5	26.5
2	7	P	1	35.0	84.0	24.5	26.0	72.0	27.0
2	7	P	2	48.5	117.0	36.0	37.0	104.0	40.0
2	7	P	3	31.0	81.5	24.0	25.5	69.0	27.0
2	7	P	4	25.5	63.5	19.5	19.0	53.0	21.5
2	7	P	5	46.0	106.5	29.5	37.5	91.5	33.5
2	7	P	6	43.5	108.0	28.5	33.5	95.0	32.5
2	8	P	1	28.0	71.0	20.0	20.5	60.0	23.5
2	8	P	2	32.0	76.5	23.5	23.5	67.5	25.0
2	8	P	3	41.5	101.5	26.5	30.0	86.5	29.5
2	8	P	4	34.0	84.0	25.0	26.0	71.5	28.0
2	8	P	5	46.0	113.5	31.0	36.5	100.0	35.5
2	8	P	6	47.0	105.0	34.0	38.5	97.0	36.5
2	9	P	1	35.0	79.5	27.5	30.0	72.0	30.0
2	9	P	2	38.0	86.0	27.0	30.0	77.5	29.0
2	9	P	3	33.0	73.0	22.5	24.0	65.0	23.5
2	9	P	4	44.0	105.0	32.5	35.5	97.0	34.5
2	9	P	5	39.5	92.5	28.5	34.5	85.0	31.5
2	9	P	6	57.0	126.0	34.5	45.5	120.0	38.0
2	10	P	1	46.0	96.0	26.5	33.5	89.0	31.0
2	10	P	2	70.5	166.0	34.5	49.0	142.0	42.0
2	10	P	3	30.0	60.5	25.5	26.0	57.0	28.0
2	10	P	4	63.0	119.5	30.0	41.0	109.0	37.5
2	10	P	5	0.0	75.5	24.5	26.0	74.0	29.0
2	10	P	6	0.0	107.0	26.0	32.0	91.5	30.5
2	1	N	1	16.0	37.0	15.0	13.5	31.0	16.0
2	1	N	2	17.5	34.0	15.0	15.0	30.0	16.5
2	2	N	1	16.0	41.0	15.0	15.0	35.0	15.5
2	2	N	2	17.0	37.5	14.5	14.5	33.0	16.5
2	3	N	1	16.0	35.5	16.5	12.5	31.0	16.5
2	3	N	2	16.5	38.0	15.0	14.0	33.0	17.0
2	4	N	1	17.0	40.0	16.0	13.5	33.0	16.5
2	4	N	2	16.5	42.0	15.0	12.5	34.0	16.0
2	5	N	1	16.0	40.5	14.5	12.5	32.5	15.0
2	5	N	2	15.5	36.0	14.5	12.5	31.0	16.0
2	6	N	1	20.0	46.0	16.5	15.0	40.5	19.5
2	6	N	2	16.0	40.0	15.0	13.0	34.5	16.5
2	7	N	1	19.0	39.0	15.0	14.0	34.0	17.0
2	7	N	2	0.0	39.0	16.0	15.0	33.5	17.5
2	8	N	1	17.0	35.5	14.0	12.5	31.5	16.0
2	8	N	2	17.5	36.5	14.0	13.0	32.0	15.0
2	9	N	1	15.5	35.0	14.5	13.5	32.0	16.0
2	9	N	2	15.5	34.0	14.5	13.0	32.0	15.0
2	10	N	1	16.0	35.5	14.5	13.0	32.5	15.0
2	10	N	2	0.0	40.0	16.5	14.0	36.0	17.5

3	1	P	1	60.5	131.0	32.4	47.4	117.0	36.5
3	1	P	2	71.3	139.0	35.6	53.1	123.0	38.0
3	1	P	3	62.2	145.5	34.2	49.3	127.6	36.0
3	1	P	4	54.5	127.2	30.6	41.7	113.6	30.7
3	1	P	5	44.7	96.7	28.7	35.5	87.5	30.2
3	1	P	6	40.5	86.6	23.0	29.2	75.7	25.0
3	2	P	1	60.8	127.0	30.2	49.4	115.4	37.5
3	2	P	2	39.8	93.8	27.5	38.7	83.8	30.5
3	2	P	3	53.7	112.2	30.0	44.7	100.5	34.1
3	2	P	4	65.2	143.0	31.8	44.2	123.1	34.2
3	2	P	5	85.8	179.0	37.5	59.0	166.7	44.2
3	2	P	6	73.3	158.8	35.6	49.4	144.4	41.1
3	3	P	1	54.1	106.4	28.5	37.0	100.5	30.5
3	3	P	2	58.5	126.9	32.0	44.0	119.0	36.4
3	3	P	3	83.5	159.8	42.0	66.8	160.0	48.3
3	3	P	4	58.5	129.0	30.3	42.0	117.5	34.9
3	3	P	5	62.0	141.2	31.0	42.2	127.2	35.0
3	3	P	6	52.6	107.5	30.0	39.1	102.5	32.9
3	4	P	1	48.9	105.5	30.5	37.4	95.0	30.8
3	4	P	2	52.4	117.4	29.6	39.4	105.0	34.1
3	4	P	3	57.8	118.6	31.8	42.5	108.4	32.9
3	4	P	4	88.0	184.8	42.9	70.4	175.0	47.0
3	4	P	5	61.2	133.5	33.3	41.5	120.0	36.2
3	4	P	6	79.9	168.7	39.1	65.8	152.1	44.4
3	5	P	1	43.6	94.4	27.0	32.1	83.8	28.5
3	5	P	2	64.4	145.4	33.7	45.3	126.5	35.9
3	5	P	3	65.0	147.2	34.6	48.5	129.5	35.4
3	5	P	4	60.6	132.5	29.4	42.8	117.6	30.7
3	5	P	5	69.0	152.8	37.3	56.1	137.4	39.5
3	5	P	6	54.4	122.8	28.4	38.6	104.9	34.2
3	6	P	1	54.0	121.5	31.2	42.0	104.7	32.3
3	6	P	2	86.5	198.2	43.1	67.1	169.4	47.2
3	6	P	3	68.1	148.7	37.7	51.1	130.9	39.9
3	6	P	4	70.2	136.4	39.7	60.9	127.3	44.9
3	6	P	5	48.2	106.4	31.4	38.3	93.6	31.1
3	6	P	6	65.9	126.3	34.5	52.3	116.0	36.2
3	7	P	1	95.8	212.0	43.7	71.0	191.4	45.0
3	7	P	2	47.6	126.0	31.1	37.6	106.4	31.5
3	7	P	3	58.2	130.9	33.5	47.6	115.2	34.7
3	7	P	4	41.1	97.9	27.6	32.6	85.0	28.5
3	7	P	5	78.5	174.3	38.1	60.0	153.7	40.5
3	7	P	6	48.7	110.0	29.8	39.1	95.2	29.9
3	8	P	1	68.7	153.0	36.0	56.5	138.8	40.2
3	8	P	2	65.1	150.2	37.9	52.2	135.7	39.4
3	8	P	3	54.0	130.5	30.4	38.5	113.8	33.0
3	8	P	4	45.0	103.1	28.4	34.8	90.5	30.6
3	8	P	5	84.0	176.6	41.2	64.4	159.7	45.3
3	8	P	6	89.9	196.6	42.9	67.3	180.7	47.5
3	9	P	1	54.7	116.3	29.2	41.1	106.9	31.5
3	9	P	2	41.4	91.5	27.1	32.3	82.8	29.6
3	9	P	3	79.9	165.9	38.1	60.0	158.0	42.0
3	9	P	4	67.0	159.6	37.5	52.7	136.4	40.2
3	9	P	5	59.4	127.7	35.4	48.6	120.0	39.4
3	9	P	6	51.4	104.0	28.8	40.2	96.2	32.4
3	10	P	1	41.0	97.0	27.0	31.6	80.8	28.4
3	10	P	2	64.5	142.5	37.5	49.5	123.2	39.5
3	10	P	3	65.2	152.5	37.0	53.1	134.6	40.2
3	10	P	4	52.2	111.2	31.1	38.1	94.7	34.0
3	10	P	5	56.3	134.3	36.2	45.7	118.6	39.9
3	10	P	6	72.9	164.2	37.9	54.3	143.5	41.4
3	1	N	1	19.1	41.4	16.6	14.0	36.0	17.6
3	1	N	2	17.4	39.2	17.3	16.2	34.3	17.1
3	2	N	1	18.8	39.9	16.4	15.7	36.0	17.2
3	2	N	2	18.4	41.0	15.7	14.1	35.9	16.7
3	3	N	1	18.0	41.5	16.3	14.4	36.5	18.0
3	3	N	2	20.5	44.0	16.9	15.5	40.0	17.9
3	4	N	1	19.7	41.6	16.9	14.5	37.3	17.3
3	4	N	2	17.0	37.9	16.4	14.4	33.2	16.9
3	5	N	1	19.0	44.0	17.2	15.2	39.2	17.8
3	5	N	2	18.0	39.8	17.6	15.5	35.3	17.4
3	6	N	1	19.5	44.5	18.5	15.3	37.6	17.8
3	6	N	2	17.3	37.5	15.6	14.9	33.1	16.1
3	7	N	1	17.6	40.5	16.7	14.0	35.0	16.8
3	7	N	2	18.6	44.3	18.4	16.4	37.8	18.2
3	8	N	1	17.9	39.6	16.6	14.4	34.8	17.7
3	8	N	2	19.4	40.3	16.5	15.4	36.0	17.1
3	9	N	1	18.4	42.0	17.6	15.1	37.5	17.5
3	9	N	2	19.4	43.0	17.0	15.3	38.4	17.1
3	10	N	1	19.0	41.1	16.4	15.4	35.1	16.1
3	10	N	2	19.3	47.3	18.4	16.1	40.5	19.1

4	1	P	1	36.3	87.3	26.1	29.2	71.1	27.3
4	1	P	2	52.0	120.6	34.0	43.2	100.7	38.2
4	1	P	3	179.8	311.5	63.2	111.6	279.1	92.2
4	1	P	4	145.2	246.1	56.4	115.6	238.0	88.1
4	1	P	5	60.8	117.0	30.9	41.0	107.0	37.1
4	1	P	6	44.4	112.2	28.2	38.1	97.4	31.2
4	2	P	1	58.2	142.3	32.3	41.0	118.2	36.5
4	2	P	2	69.0	159.8	40.0	55.2	132.6	46.8
4	2	P	3	46.1	105.0	29.1	33.1	90.9	35.3
4	2	P	4	64.1	145.4	35.5	47.6	128.6	40.1
4	2	P	5	43.8	109.1	32.9	43.0	94.4	40.0
4	2	P	6	43.0	104.0	31.5	36.6	81.3	37.9
4	3	P	1	61.4	128.6	33.1	44.1	113.8	36.2
4	3	P	2	42.2	88.5	23.1	32.5	80.8	34.7
4	3	P	3	54.2	124.5	31.3	38.5	109.2	34.9
4	3	P	4	26.2	56.0	27.1	26.1	49.4	28.7
4	3	P	5	52.2	137.5	32.6	41.7	109.6	37.7
4	3	P	6	38.8	87.2	27.1	29.9	73.2	28.9
4	4	P	1	39.1	87.7	27.5	28.6	75.6	30.5
4	4	P	2	38.6	89.1	27.1	30.4	77.4	30.5
4	4	P	3	78.0	158.5	44.3	60.6	147.2	56.4
4	4	P	4	34.6	86.2	26.5	29.5	73.3	27.1
4	4	P	5	45.9	97.7	27.5	32.9	85.6	29.1
4	4	P	6	44.1	99.9	28.5	32.3	86.4	31.8
4	5	P	1	93.5	179.0	46.4	67.2	167.3	54.8
4	5	P	2	31.8	70.9	23.2	26.1	59.2	25.1
4	5	P	3	61.2	131.4	34.6	43.8	110.0	41.8
4	5	P	4	150.3	283.2	68.8	119.0	281.4	95.8
4	5	P	5	101.2	212.5	48.2	73.2	192.3	57.9
4	5	P	6	43.8	95.8	30.5	36.7	85.2	35.1
4	6	P	1	35.1	76.8	22.8	25.0	67.5	24.6
4	6	P	2	86.9	176.9	45.4	65.7	163.8	54.6
4	6	P	3	23.6	48.4	18.4	18.5	42.6	20.1
4	6	P	4	144.2	254.1	60.9	116.2	267.7	80.7
4	6	P	5	34.0	80.4	25.4	25.8	70.5	25.8
4	6	P	6	41.6	84.8	27.1	32.3	76.4	30.3
4	7	P	1	31.8	71.5	22.3	24.7	62.5	25.9
4	7	P	2	78.0	170.8	40.3	63.2	150.3	50.2
4	7	P	3	48.3	107.7	29.4	37.1	93.9	31.2
4	7	P	4	25.5	56.5	23.2	24.6	52.5	25.0
4	7	P	5	33.0	77.1	26.0	28.4	70.1	27.2
4	7	P	6	78.4	182.6	46.2	75.6	167.0	60.0
4	1	N	1	16.2	33.4	15.8	15.1	30.9	16.2
4	1	N	2	17.6	37.3	16.0	15.2	32.5	16.1
4	2	N	1	16.2	34.0	15.6	13.4	29.6	15.8
4	2	N	2	18.6	43.9	16.9	15.5	37.2	17.8
4	3	N	1	16.2	38.2	15.1	14.1	33.0	16.4
4	3	N	2	18.0	40.1	16.6	16.0	34.9	16.9
4	4	N	1	17.6	38.8	16.4	14.2	38.1	16.7
4	4	N	2	17.4	40.9	16.0	14.6	34.9	16.8
4	5	N	1	17.1	35.7	16.3	14.6	31.3	15.9
4	5	N	2	16.3	37.0	15.8	14.7	32.8	17.0
4	6	N	1	18.0	42.2	16.2	15.8	35.2	17.6
4	6	N	2	17.1	37.5	15.8	15.0	33.2	17.0
4	7	N	1	18.8	47.0	18.0	16.4	40.1	18.2
4	7	N	2	16.1	38.1	15.1	15.3	33.4	16.4

5	1	P	1	38.5	88.0	24.5	27.5	74.0	26.5
5	1	P	2	38.0	104.0	27.5	31.0	87.5	29.0
5	1	P	3	82.0	199.0	41.0	64.5	184.0	49.0
5	1	P	4	65.0	133.0	37.5	45.0	123.0	42.5
5	1	P	5	37.0	90.0	23.5	26.5	79.0	27.5
5	1	P	6	131.0	273.0	47.5	76.5	276.0	62.0
5	2	P	1	68.0	147.5	36.0	55.0	136.0	44.5
5	2	P	2	56.0	118.0	33.0	46.5	107.0	44.5
5	2	P	3	34.5	82.0	24.0	28.5	73.0	27.5
5	2	P	4	49.5	122.0	30.0	46.0	100.0	37.5
5	2	P	5	45.0	106.0	27.0	33.0	89.0	32.0
5	2	P	6	19.5	44.0	15.7	15.5	39.0	17.0
5	3	P	1	56.5	122.0	35.5	46.0	112.0	41.5
5	3	P	2	65.0	142.0	38.5	56.0	134.0	51.0
5	3	P	3	29.5	67.5	22.0	29.5	60.0	25.0
5	3	P	4	115.0	232.0	46.0	78.0	224.0	60.0
5	3	P	5	40.5	82.5	22.5	29.5	74.0	26.0
5	3	P	6	55.0	129.0	32.0	41.0	109.0	36.5
5	4	P	1	91.0	225.0	41.5	63.0	187.0	49.5
5	4	P	2	35.0	102.0	27.0	29.5	77.0	28.5
5	4	P	3	51.5	136.0	33.0	40.0	107.0	38.0
5	4	P	4	26.5	71.0	20.5	20.5	54.5	21.0
5	4	P	5	54.5	150.0	30.0	43.0	110.0	35.5
5	4	P	6	47.0	136.0	29.5	37.0	96.5	33.0
5	5	P	1	46.0	102.0	35.5	44.5	94.5	41.0
5	5	P	2	56.0	98.0	30.0	42.5	89.0	35.0
5	5	P	3	59.0	128.0	31.0	44.5	114.0	33.5
5	5	P	4	75.0	187.0	39.0	58.0	163.0	49.0
5	5	P	5	35.0	72.5	24.5	28.5	65.5	27.0
5	5	P	6	48.5	126.0	32.0	39.0	116.0	37.0
5	6	P	1	26.5	66.0	21.5	20.5	55.0	22.5
5	6	P	2	59.5	141.0	32.0	46.5	124.0	41.0
5	6	P	3	66.5	160.0	33.0	59.0	136.5	45.0
5	6	P	4	27.5	68.0	19.5	21.0	53.5	23.0
5	6	P	5	63.0	157.0	37.0	56.0	135.0	48.0
5	6	P	6	55.0	134.0	30.0	44.0	57.5	39.5
5	1	N	1	17.5	37.5	15.0	13.0	35.0	15.0
5	1	N	2	16.5	38.5	15.5	13.5	33.0	15.0
5	2	N	1	16.5	41.0	16.0	13.2	36.0	16.5
5	2	N	2	16.8	39.5	15.0	13.5	33.5	15.0
5	3	N	1	16.0	39.5	17.0	14.2	35.5	17.0
5	3	N	2	17.0	35.0	14.2	13.0	30.0	15.0
5	4	N	1	18.5	53.0	17.5	15.5	41.0	19.0
5	4	N	2	18.5	47.0	16.0	13.5	35.5	17.5
5	5	N	1	18.0	41.5	18.0	15.5	36.0	17.5
5	5	N	2	18.0	38.0	16.0	15.0	34.5	16.5
5	6	N	1	15.5	37.0	15.0	14.0	32.5	16.0
5	6	N	2	15.0	40.0	14.0	12.5	32.0	15.0

6	1	P	1	202.5	334.0	77.7	134.0	276.0	111.7
6	1	P	2	70.0	144.0	36.5	58.1	127.7	47.3
6	1	P	3	50.2	94.2	34.2	45.4	82.0	39.5
6	1	P	4	155.0	213.0	54.0	87.0	196.2	68.8
6	1	P	5	25.0	56.7	0.0	20.0	45.5	22.0
6	1	P	6	58.0	122.5	39.5	57.2	111.0	46.5
6	2	P	1	53.5	115.5	30.5	44.0	103.5	36.5
6	2	P	2	86.5	176.0	51.5	79.2	171.8	74.0
6	2	P	3	64.8	133.5	38.2	54.5	120.0	47.8
6	2	P	4	67.5	142.0	43.8	69.6	132.5	58.5
6	2	P	5	79.1	175.0	40.0	63.5	158.5	50.7
6	2	P	6	54.8	114.5	33.0	57.5	107.5	39.5
6	3	P	1	56.5	112.5	33.0	42.2	98.4	36.0
6	3	P	2	73.0	137.4	41.2	56.8	126.8	46.8
6	3	P	3	66.0	132.5	39.0	49.4	118.5	44.5
6	3	P	4	116.5	210.5	55.8	86.5	188.5	69.4
6	3	P	5	55.0	109.8	35.0	48.7	97.8	42.5
6	3	P	6	100.0	190.0	45.0	73.7	166.0	53.8
6	4	P	1	132.8	277.5	60.2	104.5	259.5	85.5
6	4	P	2	73.5	153.0	39.2	66.0	133.0	48.6
6	4	P	3	51.6	123.0	32.2	38.3	103.7	39.2
6	4	P	4	80.7	172.0	41.7	62.0	149.0	49.0
6	4	P	5	116.5	228.0	50.3	91.5	200.0	69.0
6	4	P	6	68.8	145.6	36.1	55.6	125.6	47.2
6	5	P	1	70.5	143.5	38.6	55.0	133.5	43.5
6	5	P	2	48.0	124.7	30.4	35.0	99.6	34.8
6	5	P	3	64.2	124.5	39.8	57.4	120.0	48.9
6	5	P	4	53.4	113.7	32.5	40.7	100.5	35.3
6	5	P	5	85.2	178.8	42.0	65.5	156.6	49.7
6	5	P	6	48.4	100.2	27.5	37.1	90.0	31.0
6	6	P	1	77.0	164.5	43.4	70.5	157.3	56.8
6	6	P	2	74.0	163.2	39.5	53.0	147.7	43.0
6	6	P	3	54.5	105.0	33.0	35.0	101.5	33.0
6	6	P	4	222.0	412.0	98.2	155.0	382.0	153.2
6	6	P	5	65.5	151.8	38.7	51.2	131.0	52.6
6	6	P	6	61.6	124.7	38.2	48.5	114.2	42.3
6	7	P	1	48.0	122.9	34.3	39.1	104.6	36.5
6	7	P	2	96.0	196.6	43.7	62.8	185.4	53.8
6	7	P	3	72.7	152.5	37.2	47.0	136.4	43.7
6	7	P	4	81.5	161.6	41.8	59.0	146.4	50.5
6	7	P	5	87.2	169.0	40.0	56.0	156.5	46.5
6	7	P	6	67.5	133.5	35.8	46.0	124.0	39.8
6	8	P	1	158.3	291.5	62.0	106.5	281.5	86.8
6	8	P	2	55.6	137.9	29.2	45.0	112.2	35.4
6	8	P	3	54.0	108.5	31.5	42.8	95.4	35.9
6	8	P	4	97.5	211.0	51.4	75.9	186.2	72.1
6	8	P	5	55.9	109.5	32.5	42.8	95.2	35.1
6	8	P	6	45.0	86.6	28.8	39.8	75.4	39.4
6	9	P	1	57.1	112.8	37.0	47.7	102.5	38.2
6	9	P	2	70.8	150.6	38.5	52.5	126.6	40.1
6	9	P	3	46.4	98.8	40.0	50.0	89.8	41.0
6	9	P	4	40.1	93.4	31.2	34.8	82.3	32.5
6	9	P	5	28.5	63.4	22.5	25.5	54.5	24.4
6	9	P	6	56.6	125.4	34.7	48.0	110.2	39.6
6	10	P	1	84.0	175.5	36.7	57.7	149.6	47.4
6	10	P	2	46.7	98.0	28.3	36.0	84.0	29.5
6	10	P	3	45.8	105.6	29.1	34.5	87.2	35.0
6	10	P	4	92.9	191.8	43.5	83.9	166.4	57.8
6	10	P	5	93.7	202.6	50.8	88.0	183.8	66.5
6	10	P	6	55.4	116.5	25.2	41.1	99.0	32.4
6	1	N	1	19.5	41.2	16.5	15.5	36.5	18.5
6	1	N	2	21.0	50.0	19.5	17.0	41.8	22.3
6	2	N	1	18.0	41.0	16.5	15.0	36.5	18.0
6	2	N	2	17.8	41.4	15.8	14.5	35.4	17.4
6	3	N	1	21.0	45.5	17.0	15.5	40.0	17.8
6	3	N	2	19.5	43.0	16.7	15.9	37.5	17.0
6	4	N	1	19.7	50.0	19.8	16.7	40.5	19.8
6	4	N	2	18.5	42.5	16.2	14.7	35.5	16.8
6	5	N	1	20.9	47.5	19.5	16.9	42.0	19.5
6	5	N	2	20.4	48.0	18.0	17.0	44.0	19.5
6	6	N	1	19.0	46.0	17.6	15.2	39.1	17.7
6	6	N	2	18.0	40.0	16.7	13.9	36.8	16.7
6	7	N	1	20.0	47.7	16.7	14.9	42.7	17.7
6	7	N	2	21.0	44.7	17.8	17.0	38.6	19.2
6	8	N	1	17.1	40.9	17.5	15.0	37.0	18.0
6	8	N	2	19.7	52.9	19.4	16.7	44.3	21.1
6	9	N	1	16.4	37.0	15.8	13.4	33.4	16.5
6	9	N	2	17.7	45.5	18.0	15.8	38.8	17.8
6	10	N	1	21.5	57.0	19.9	17.7	46.5	20.8
6	10	N	2	17.7	42.2	15.6	14.4	34.4	16.8

7	1	P	1	67.8	141.8	35.2	48.2	119.2	41.8
7	1	P	2	74.0	161.8	38.8	53.5	138.6	44.8
7	1	P	3	49.8	111.2	29.8	35.0	91.8	31.6
7	1	P	4	44.8	164.5	30.8	38.0	92.4	33.8
7	1	?	5	92.2	171.8	42.4	67.8	162.0	48.0
7	1	P	6	95.6	197.0	41.8	66.8	176.8	46.0
7	2	P	1	57.0	122.8	33.2	44.2	111.2	40.8
7	2	P	2	51.2	109.6	31.6	37.7	100.7	39.6
7	2	P	3	38.2	86.8	28.8	33.4	79.2	32.6
7	2	P	4	72.8	145.6	37.5	54.2	138.8	48.0
7	2	P	5	53.2	120.4	28.2	38.4	109.0	33.4
7	2	P	6	31.8	70.4	23.4	25.5	64.6	26.8
7	3	P	1	91.2	168.4	41.5	59.0	149.2	44.2
7	3	P	2	94.7	173.0	38.6	57.8	150.4	47.6
7	3	P	3	61.2	116.8	33.0	40.8	104.9	38.3
7	3	P	4	58.2	122.0	29.4	36.4	106.2	33.8
7	3	P	5	28.2	64.4	21.0	19.4	54.0	22.2
7	3	P	6	56.4	113.2	31.3	38.5	94.8	34.8
7	4	P	1	67.4	158.4	34.8	49.5	132.6	40.8
7	4	P	2	53.5	122.8	28.6	37.6	99.6	31.5
7	4	P	3	58.6	121.8	31.2	41.0	102.6	36.2
7	4	P	4	65.5	145.2	32.8	48.0	123.2	38.4
7	4	P	5	52.5	115.0	26.4	35.8	101.2	29.8
7	4	P	6	36.4	78.4	21.8	24.8	66.5	24.5
7	5	P	1	49.5	127.4	30.0	35.2	113.8	32.4
7	5	P	2	43.3	101.2	27.8	29.0	91.2	27.6
7	5	P	3	39.2	94.8	27.8	29.9	83.2	28.5
7	5	P	4	37.0	92.2	32.2	28.2	81.2	27.6
7	5	P	5	51.2	110.8	30.2	35.6	96.8	31.4
7	5	P	6	61.5	123.8	38.8	48.3	116.4	42.2
7	6	P	1	83.2	163.4	48.8	60.6	161.8	47.8
7	6	P	2	38.3	84.2	25.4	28.6	70.8	24.2
7	6	P	3	34.6	70.0	22.8	23.2	61.8	22.6
7	6	P	4	32.5	71.8	25.2	24.4	59.6	23.8
7	6	P	5	33.8	75.8	23.4	25.4	60.8	22.2
7	6	P	6	31.0	68.8	23.8	25.1	65.4	24.0
7	7	P	1	71.2	149.8	37.8	54.3	127.7	42.5
7	7	P	2	56.4	124.2	30.2	40.8	107.2	34.1
7	7	P	3	49.4	109.1	26.9	37.0	92.5	29.1
7	7	P	4	49.2	118.4	29.1	37.1	94.2	31.8
7	7	P	5	39.6	79.6	25.5	30.5	69.2	27.8
7	7	P	6	51.8	130.8	32.6	42.7	110.5	36.6
7	8	P	1	40.0	88.8	26.8	30.1	75.0	29.2
7	8	P	2	44.4	113.2	27.6	31.9	90.6	31.8
7	8	P	3	85.1	167.0	43.8	66.4	157.8	53.4
7	8	P	4	66.0	139.4	36.5	49.5	121.5	39.5
7	8	P	5	72.4	162.0	33.5	46.4	130.0	35.5
7	8	P	6	48.7	102.2	30.2	40.1	88.2	32.8
7	9	P	1	33.8	75.4	24.6	25.5	66.8	25.4
7	9	P	2	39.1	87.8	28.3	33.0	81.8	32.1
7	9	P	3	116.8	119.0	30.2	43.0	103.7	33.5
7	9	P	4	41.5	92.1	26.2	30.1	77.6	29.1
7	9	P	5	58.8	145.2	35.3	50.8	128.3	41.9
7	9	P	6	48.6	100.4	29.2	34.0	87.5	31.7
7	10	P	1	52.3	121.6	28.8	37.0	102.1	31.0
7	10	P	2	85.5	173.6	38.5	59.1	158.2	45.2
7	10	P	3	62.4	130.0	31.5	43.8	111.8	35.0
7	10	P	4	56.0	126.1	28.1	38.7	108.7	31.9
7	10	P	5	49.4	104.5	27.2	32.5	92.5	29.2
7	10	P	6	88.0	167.9	36.4	56.8	151.0	43.4
7	1	N	1	24.8	49.6	18.2	17.0	45.4	16.5
7	1	N	2	21.8	40.2	15.0	14.8	36.6	14.8
7	2	N	1	16.6	38.6	13.8	14.4	34.2	15.2
7	2	N	2	18.6	42.6	16.5	14.6	37.7	17.0
7	3	N	1	17.0	38.6	15.8	13.6	33.8	16.4
7	3	N	2	20.0	48.4	17.6	16.2	41.4	19.2
7	4	N	1	17.0	42.2	14.6	13.2	34.8	15.8
7	4	N	2	20.8	50.6	16.6	16.2	45.5	17.6
7	5	N	1	18.4	46.7	16.5	13.4	41.2	16.2
7	5	N	2	17.0	43.8	15.6	13.0	38.0	15.5
7	6	N	1	16.0	47.6	14.2	13.2	36.4	14.4
7	6	N	2	17.5	38.5	14.6	14.4	34.0	15.2
7	7	N	1	15.8	36.1	13.9	13.2	31.6	15.2
7	7	N	2	16.0	34.4	14.0	13.0	33.5	15.0
7	8	N	1	17.8	41.8	15.6	13.9	35.8	16.4
7	8	N	2	18.0	45.0	15.8	14.6	37.2	16.2
7	9	N	1	18.9	46.8	16.4	15.1	41.0	16.6
7	9	N	2	17.6	45.0	15.1	13.0	34.2	14.4
7	10	N	1	18.3	43.7	15.2	13.8	37.7	15.8
7	10	N	2	21.5	49.4	17.8	16.6	41.9	19.8

8	2	P	1	60.2	131.2	36.0	42.3	118.6	39.1
8	2	P	2	59.1	122.0	36.0	53.0	118.4	40.7
8	2	P	3	53.2	115.0	34.0	40.7	105.4	39.0
8	2	P	4	83.4	188.0	43.7	56.2	175.5	48.2
8	2	P	5	56.2	123.7	33.3	40.5	112.8	38.1
8	2	P	6	27.6	58.4	21.1	20.3	53.0	23.9
8	3	P	2	69.6	144.6	38.1	55.5	137.0	46.0
8	3	P	3	35.0	70.6	24.6	27.1	64.5	28.4
8	3	P	4	71.5	135.6	36.0	51.1	127.6	44.0
8	3	P	5	70.0	136.8	38.4	53.4	134.8	45.6
8	3	P	6	68.8	143.8	37.0	61.7	131.1	43.8
8	4	P	1	75.6	170.0	40.5	58.8	154.2	50.1
8	4	P	2	39.2	155.8	29.1	32.3	0.0	30.8
8	4	P	3	51.8	171.4	31.9	40.3	99.0	35.2
8	4	P	5	67.4	153.4	38.4	56.2	134.6	43.0
8	5	P	2	84.0	163.2	44.8	66.8	165.5	50.8
8	5	P	3	58.2	122.0	43.8	53.6	118.5	46.7
8	5	P	4	80.8	143.6	43.7	62.4	144.2	58.0
8	5	P	5	82.6	163.7	46.4	59.8	163.8	51.6
8	6	P	4	60.4	124.4	38.3	50.1	118.2	42.8
8	2	N	1	19.5	39.2	17.2	14.0	35.2	17.5
8	2	N	2	19.4	42.7	17.4	14.2	37.2	17.5
8	3	N	1	18.4	41.6	16.3	15.1	36.3	16.0
8	3	N	2	18.5	40.0	15.0	13.4	36.0	17.0
8	4	N	1	17.5	37.6	14.8	14.2	33.0	15.8
8	4	N	2	17.4	40.2	16.2	14.4	34.4	16.2
8	5	N	1	17.0	40.7	15.3	12.4	34.9	15.0
8	5	N	2	19.0	43.8	16.9	14.1	38.8	17.1
8	6	N	1	16.3	36.1	14.0	12.0	32.0	15.2
8	6	N	2	16.4	33.4	14.0	13.1	30.1	14.1
9	1	P	1	52.8	91.9	28.5	33.9	84.5	30.5
9	1	P	2	54.3	125.9	33.4	38.9	115.9	37.4
9	1	P	3	30.0	68.5	23.0	23.0	56.2	23.8
9	1	P	6	29.0	56.8	24.2	21.9	68.2	25.0
9	2	P	1	47.2	120.0	32.2	37.8	95.8	33.7
9	2	P	2	60.0	133.0	38.4	49.7	111.5	43.8
9	2	P	5	45.2	98.4	30.0	37.4	82.0	33.0
9	3	P	1	47.3	128.4	32.8	37.0	103.0	42.8
9	3	P	2	49.3	113.0	34.5	39.4	96.0	38.2
9	3	P	3	44.2	53.8	29.0	32.2	90.6	31.5
9	3	P	4	66.1	164.5	40.6	52.5	132.7	49.4
9	3	P	6	40.0	53.0	42.4	32.4	89.6	38.0
9	4	P	1	64.5	145.6	34.7	46.9	128.1	43.1
9	4	P	2	70.5	154.3	37.6	50.7	137.6	44.3
9	4	P	4	33.6	77.1	25.8	24.7	65.6	28.8
9	4	P	5	43.9	96.8	28.1	35.4	0.0	33.0
9	4	P	6	45.0	103.1	30.2	36.1	96.0	34.7
9	5	P	1	59.1	127.3	33.9	39.7	114.3	40.0
9	5	P	2	81.5	173.7	41.5	0.0	175.3	49.7
9	5	P	5	50.0	100.8	32.0	38.1	97.5	34.8
9	6	P	1	60.5	127.0	37.1	46.0	113.6	37.8
9	6	P	2	71.2	146.1	37.5	51.6	134.6	40.9
9	6	P	4	86.7	202.0	46.2	72.0	184.9	54.3
9	6	P	5	39.1	92.3	27.0	31.4	81.2	30.1
9	6	P	6	50.6	49.0	34.0	39.1	0.0	37.4
9	1	N	1	21.4	44.5	17.1	18.0	38.0	18.2
9	1	N	2	18.2	38.4	18.0	14.2	42.3	17.9
9	2	N	2	19.2	44.6	16.4	15.2	36.6	18.2
9	3	N	1	19.0	39.4	17.2	15.0	37.9	18.4
9	3	N	2	18.2	41.3	16.6	16.0	35.2	19.4
9	4	N	1	18.1	45.4	16.5	15.0	39.3	17.8
9	4	N	2	17.7	37.3	15.9	13.3	33.3	17.4
9	5	N	1	18.0	33.3	19.6	21.9	34.0	19.0
9	5	N	2	17.7	34.5	16.1	14.5	33.0	16.3
9	6	N	1	17.8	47.3	15.3	15.0	37.1	17.9
9	6	N	2	19.8	41.0	17.4	16.2	37.3	17.5

10	1	P	1	36.7	80.5	23.5	24.5	80.0	21.7
10	1	P	2	29.1	73.3	22.2	25.0	64.9	25.0
10	1	P	3	53.9	132.1	33.7	58.0	122.0	39.2
10	1	P	4	31.1	78.5	22.0	21.0	67.4	23.9
10	1	P	5	28.2	66.8	22.7	24.3	59.2	25.8
10	2	P	3	73.6	169.9	38.3	61.0	169.5	44.5
10	2	P	5	34.0	97.5	26.7	29.5	85.5	28.4
10	2	P	6	37.6	96.0	25.1	29.1	83.3	27.0
10	3	P	4	36.2	92.8	24.7	31.1	77.3	29.7
10	3	P	5	48.8	122.0	28.1	39.3	107.9	34.0
10	2	P	6	33.8	86.3	24.1	27.9	76.7	29.1
10	4	P	1	53.5	126.5	33.4	43.0	116.0	36.7
10	4	P	2	48.0	131.5	30.3	35.4	102.3	33.7
10	4	P	3	67.9	198.3	46.7	62.4	184.6	50.4
10	4	P	4	51.9	145.1	32.0	42.1	128.4	38.2
10	4	P	6	53.4	143.1	32.8	40.6	116.6	36.7
10	5	P	2	46.5	117.8	28.0	41.4	100.3	31.8
10	5	P	3	30.2	75.9	23.1	26.1	66.1	26.1
10	6	P	1	77.3	189.0	39.1	64.0	163.1	44.1
10	6	P	3	27.0	65.6	21.3	20.9	58.0	21.5
10	6	P	4	65.0	159.5	38.8	59.1	161.7	43.5
10	6	P	5	66.6	181.9	36.7	52.2	154.7	41.2
10	1	N	1	15.3	32.8	14.2	12.2	30.2	14.6
10	1	N	2	18.3	50.4	15.7	15.0	40.3	19.0
10	2	N	1	18.8	46.4	18.6	17.2	38.2	19.7
10	2	N	2	17.6	0.0	16.1	15.4	38.7	17.6
10	3	N	1	16.2	39.7	16.2	13.8	34.2	17.2
10	3	N	2	18.5	44.3	16.3	16.0	37.9	17.8
10	4	N	1	16.4	41.2	15.4	13.8	35.1	15.9
10	4	N	2	17.2	39.5	14.9	14.0	32.2	16.1
10	5	N	1	17.8	38.6	14.6	13.9	33.4	15.5
10	5	N	2	18.7	43.1	16.4	14.9	36.8	16.6
10	6	N	1	16.7	40.4	14.8	13.2	34.7	14.8
10	6	N	2	18.2	43.0	15.9	15.0	37.1	16.6

Chapter 5:   A STATISTICIAN'S INDEPENDENT EVALUATION.

J.A. TOMENSON

1. INTRODUCTION

The European Community Bureau of Reference (BCR) calibration study has established the statistical basis for calibration of thromboplastins (1). Previous approaches to calibration (2,3,4) have been based on an observation by Biggs and Denson (5) that prothrombin ratios obtained with two different thromboplastins plotted against each other are distributed around a straight line passing through the point (1,1). However, the Biggs-Denson procedure was found to be inadequate in some cases and an alternative calibration model was adopted in the BCR study. A full discussion of the failings of the Biggs-Denson procedure and the arguments for proposing this alternative calibration model are given by Kirkwood (6). The new calibration procedure has now been used succesfully to calibrate three new BCR reference thromboplastins (human, bovine, and rabbit) against the WHO International Reference Preparation (IRP). It is now possible for manufacturers to calibrate their reagents against the BCR reference materials and the results of a prothrombin test may be reported as an International Normalised Ratio (INR), the theoretical ratio which would have been obtained with the IRP. The procedure has also been used successfully to calibrate the proposed second WHO IRP (BCT/253) against the existing IRP in an international collaborative exercise (7,8). In this latter exercise it was found necessary to modify the procedure in a manner to be described. Furthermore this report describes a detailed retrospective examination of the BCR calibration procedure which reveals a number of other issues which have not yet been resolved satisfactorily and merit further discussion.

The international exercise to calibrate BCT/253 was modified as a result of dropping the assumption that the separate lines for patients and normals should be coincidental. This assumption is important from the practical standpoint as it greatly simplifies the process of prothrombin ratio conversion. However, for this purpose it is sufficient to demonstrate that the mean logarithms of the prothrombin times of normals lie on the orthogonal regression line through patients' plasmas. This modification is discussed in Section 2 together with the related problem of inadequacy of the BCR calibration model. It is suggested that the calibration model needs to be generalised if it is not to suffer from a limitation similar to that of the Biggs-Denson procedure of forcing the calibration line through the point (1,1).

Confidence intervals are discussed in Section 3. It is demonstrated that the stated intervals of the BCR report are not correct. This error resulted from neglecting the variation about the calibration line. Not enough attention has been paid to the scatter about the calibration line although it is an important determinant of the usefulness of the calibration.

A further problem concerns the applicability of these calibrations to clinical practice. The BCR calibration exercise was performed using only plasma samples from stabilised patients who had undergone at least six weeks treatment. It cannot be assumed that the certified values can be used to calculate INRs for patients in the early stages of treatment or who are not stabilised. Two reference thromboplastins, the second proposed IRP and the BCR rabbit thromboplastin RBT/79 have therefore been calibrated against the widely used commercial reagent Simplastin in two separate exercises. One set of calibrations was performed using plasma from long-term stabilised patients as specified in the BCR protocol whilst the other series of calibrations were performed using patients who had undergone less than three weeks of coumarin therapy. The results are presented in Section 4.

Finally, the hierarchical scheme for calibration is discussed in Section 5. Manufacturers have been recommended to calibrate their products against BCR reference material of the same species. However, the present analysis shows that this does not necessarily achieve the best calibration results.

2. THE CALIBRATION MODEL

2.1. Adequacy of the calibration model

The new calibration method has given good results in the European (BCR) calibration exercise and an international collaborative study (1,7,8). The main assumption of the model is that the relationship between the logarithms of prothrombin times with different thromboplastins is approximately linear. This has been demonstrated empirically. An additional finding has been that the use of logarithms also achieves homoscedasticity. However, the new calibration model does have one important weakness that was apparent in both calibration studies and particularly in the study by Van den Besselaar and Van der Velde (9) in which manufacturers calibrate their products against the BCR reference materials. This is the failure in several instances of the normal control plasmas to lie on the line through patients' plasmas. An example of such a calibration is shown in Fig. 1. For the calibration to have any real practical value, it is important that this be the case as it greatly simplifies the process of converting a prothrombin ratio from one thromboplastin to another. If a single calibration equation cannot be used for both patients and normals it is still possible to relate prothrombin times of patients. This is of far less value since patients' results are now generally expressed as ratios as are therapeutic ranges. To facilitate the conversion of prothrombin ratios a more general model is required.

If the same calibration equation is valid for patients and normals it can be shown (6) that the calibration model implies a relationship between prothrombin ratios of the form

$$r_1 = r_2^b \qquad \text{(equation 1)}$$

where r_1 and r_2 are prothrombin ratios with two thromboplastins and b the slope of their calibration line. The succes of the new calibration procedure hinges on the ability of this model to

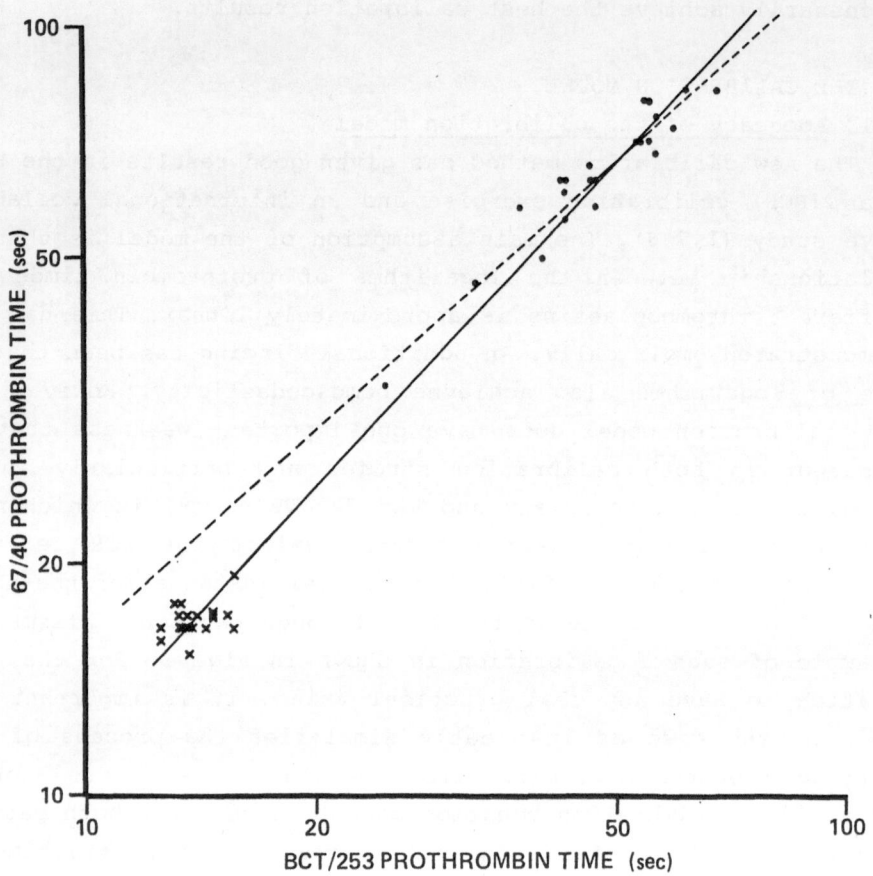

FIGURE 1. In some instances, the relationship between the logarithms of prothrombin ratios does not conform to the assumptions of the new calibration model. The plotted data points are an example where the orthogonal regression line derived from patients' plasmas does not pass through the mean of the normal control plasmas.

describe the relationship between prothrombin ratios. It should come as no surprise after previous experience with the Biggs-Denson procedure that this model will occasionally prove unsatisfactory. Fig. 2 shows this relationship for thromboplastins of differing sensitivity calibrated against the IRP. It can be seen that for ratios with the IRP in the range 1.5-5.0 the relationship is approximately linear and permits a wide variety of

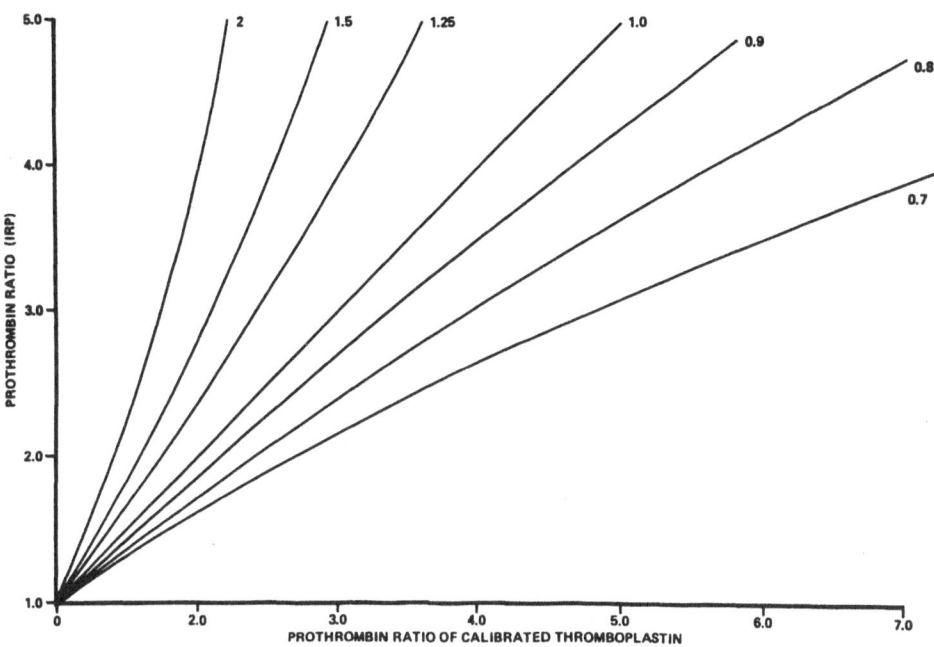

FIGURE 2. Examples are shown of the relationships used to convert prothrombin ratios into INRs for thromboplastins of differing sensitivity. The curves are of the form $y = x^b$ with the value of b given alongside each curve.

slopes. However, just as the calibration lines of the Biggs-Denson procedure were forced to pass through the point (1,1) so the intercepts of these approximate lines are also restricted. The natural way to overcome this problem is to introduce a scale parameter and use a model for prothrombin ratios of the form

$$r_1 = 10^d r_2^b \qquad \text{(equation 2)}$$

Clearly equation 1 is a particular example of equation 2 but the new model will also cope with data sets for which the mean logarithms of the prothrombin times of normals do not lie on the orthogonal regression line of the patients.

The estimation of d is made easier if a further slight modification is made to the calibration model. This is merely an as-

sumption that the prothrombin times of normal control plasmas
should each follow the same distribution rather than having separate individual distributions as is currently assumed. With this
assumption it can be shown that d is estimated as

$$d = \bar{y}_n - a - b\bar{x}_n \qquad \text{(equation 3)}$$

where $\bar{x}_n$, $\bar{y}_n$ are the mean logarithms of the prothrombin
times of normals and a, b the slope and intercept of the orthogonal regression line calculated using only the results of patients. This is the natural estimate of d and it has already been
used in (9) to provide a conversion formula for prothrombin ratios when a single calibration equation could not be used for
patients and normals.

2.2. Testing for adequacy of the calibration model

In the BCR study an assumption was made that a single straight
line describes the relationship between logarithms of the prothrombin times of both normals and patients and a test made for
coincidence of the separate lines derived using only the data
from patients or normals. If this examination of the data reveals
no statistical differences between the lines it is justifiable to
describe the relationship by a single line based on the combined
patients' and normals' data. It has already been noted that this
is an important test as it indicates whether equation 1 is a
valid formula for the conversion of prothrombin ratios. However,
for this purpose it is not neccesary to make such a stringent
assumption and it can be misleading. It is not reasonable to
expect the plasmas of normal controls to follow the same relationship since there are major biological differences between
patient and normal plasmas. More importantly the relationship
observed for normal plasmas may simply result from correlation
between the measurement errors. A hypothetical demonstration of
this point is given in Fig.3. The distributions of the points
about the calibration lines are represented by a series of ellipses. These individual deviations from the straight line are determined by biological variation and measurement error. If they
are correlated it is unlikely that the relationship between nor-

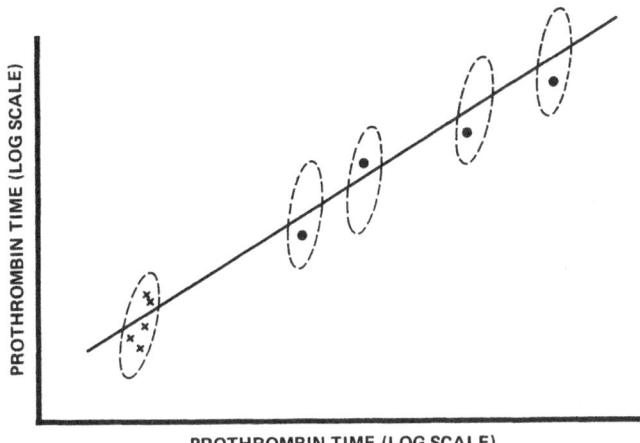

FIGURE 3. The distributions of individual deviations from the calibration line are represented by ellipses. The sign of the correlation between the individual deviations is denoted by the orientation of the ellipse and the strength of the correlation by its elongation. The example shows how correlation between the deviations from the calibration line can result in a different relationship for normal controls to that of the overall calibration line.

mal plasmas will be the same as the overall calibration line.

For equation 1 to be used in a conversion formula for prothrombin ratios it is sufficient to demonstrate that the mean logarithms of the prothrombin times of normals lie on the orthogonal regression line through patients' plasmas. A test of this hypothesis can alternatively be regarded as a test that $d = 0$ in equation 2. The use of equation 2 enables a more logical approach to be made to calibration of thromboplastins. The first step is to fit a model of the form specified by equation 2 which amounts to deriving the orthogonal regression line for patients' plasmas and estimating d by use of equation 3. A test can then be made of the hypothesis that $d = 0$ and an approximate test of this hypothesis is given in the Appendix. If the scale parameter is not significantly different from unity, the simpler equation 1 may

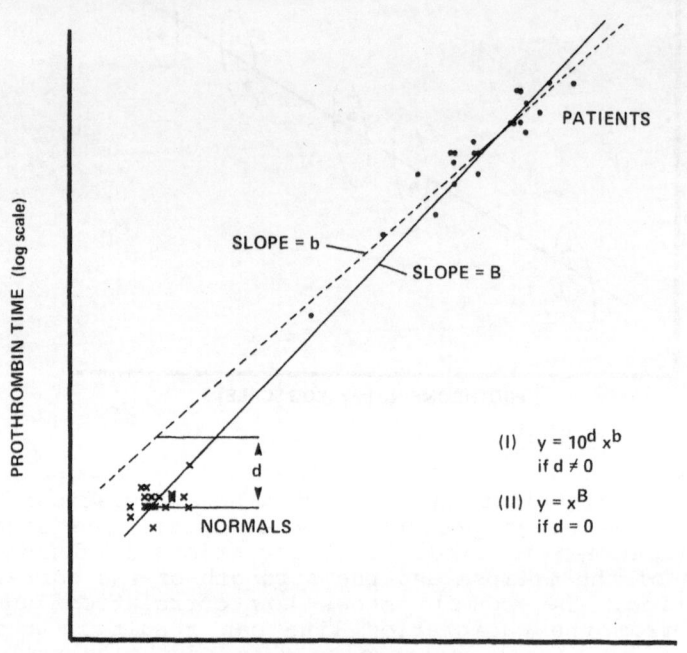

FIGURE 4. In the revised calibration procedure a test is made of the hypothesis that the mean logarithms of the prothrombin times of normals lie on the orthogonal regression line of patients' plasmas. If this hypothesis is rejected the vertical distance of the mean logarithms of the normal prothrombin times from the line (d) is incorporated in the conversion formula for prothrombin ratios.

be used and calibration proceeds in the usual manner. The procedure is illustrated in Fig. 4.

The modification of the calibration procedure is in essence little more than a formal rendering of the pragmatic approach adopted in (9). The results of the European (BCR) calibration exercise, the international collaborative study and the Manufacturers calibration study (1,7,8,9) suggest that the generalised model will rarely be needed. For most calibrations the mean logarithms of the prothrombin times of normals do lie on the orthogonal regression line through patients' plasmas. Nevertheless, it is important that clear guidelines should be available in the event that the assumptions of the calibration model are not satisfied.

3. CONFIDENCE INTERVALS

Once it has been demonstrated that the calibration model is a good description of the data, the most important parameter is not the slope of the calibration line but the variation about the line. This is the factor which will determine whether the calibration has any practical value. An INR is merely a guide to the prothrombin ratio that would have been obtained if the IRP had been used. Such estimates are valueless without an indication of their precision.

Although confidence intervals were provided in the BCR study the stated values are not correct. The confidence intervals in the report are those for the orthogonal regression estimate and reflect only the precision of the estimate of the average relationship between thromboplastins. These are not the correct intervals to be used for individual patients' ratios and times. The confidence interval that should be used is one which allows for the fact that a future individual observation will be distributed randomly about the predicted point on the calibration line. This is directly analogous to the case of ordinary linear regression where the confidence interval used for a regression estimate is different from that for a predicted future individual observation. The stated interval does not reflect the real uncertainty in the INR. Table 1 shows the actual distribution of data from the seven European laboratories in the BCR study in relation to the stated 95% confidence intervals for prothrombin times. The confidence intervals are for prothrombin times with IRP corresponding to prothrombin times obtained with each of the BCR reference materials and the other WHO reference thromboplastins. The percentage of observations contained by the intervals ranges from 32% to 55%, considerably less than the expected 95%.

Table 1. The percentages of patients and normals lying within the stated 95% confidence intervals for prothrombin times with the IRP.

	calibrated thromboplastin				
	70/178	68/434	BCT/099	RBT/79	OBT/79
patients	52.6	32.6	49.9	52.9	41.7
normals	61.3	31.5	48.4	50.8	30.6
overall	55.0	32.3	49.5	52.4	38.7

The uncertainty in an estimate of the slope of the calibration line and the standard deviation about it are dependent on the use to which it is put. Inter-laboratory differences in calibration relationships must be considered if a calibration line is to be used outside the laboratory where it was derived. The effect on the size of confidence intervals for INRs can be marked, particularly if a number of steps are involved in the calibration. The calibration of RBT/79 against the IRP in the BCR study can be used to illustrate the difference in error. For this calibration the average standard error of the estimated slope of the calibration line was 0.038 which represents the average degree of uncertainty if the calibration is used "in house". However, the standard deviation of the estimated slope between laboratories is 0.096 which represents the uncertainty in the calibration line if applied outside the laboratory at which it was derived. The magnitude of the inter-laboratory variation of the slope of the calibration line is not known. However, the BCR study and the international collaborative exercise to calibrate BCT/253 suggest a coefficient of variation (CV) of the order of 5 per cent. This uncertainty can be reduced by estimating the calibration relationship from the results of several laboratories as has been done in the two collaborative exercises (1,7). This is unlikely to be the case when manufacturers calibrate their own products.

The biggest errors are likely to occur in the calibrated values for rabbit thromboplastin. Manufacturers are recommended to calibrate a house standard against the BCR rabbit thromboplastin RBT/79 and then calibrate production lots against the house standard. The cumulative inaccuracy for such a calibration is not known but it will depend on the correlation between the two calibration steps involved in the calibration of a production lot against the BCR rabbit thromboplastin. The BCR study has shown that there is a strong correlation between the results of different calibrations performed within the same laboratory. Hermans et al (10) report the slopes of the orthogonal regression lines for the calibration of the BCR reference materials and the secondary WHO IRPs against the primary IRP obtained by each of the ten laboratories in the BCR study. The correlation between the calibration lines of the WHO and BCR rabbit thromboplastins is 0.78 and 0.89 for the WHO and BCR bovine thromboplastins. If a CV of 5% is assumed for each of the two calibration steps, house standard against production lot and house standard against the BCR rabbit thromboplastin, a CV of between 7 and 10 per cent will result for the combined calibration. This figure is dependent on the strength of the correlation between the two calibrations and the results of the BCR study indicate a CV much closer to 10 per cent than 7 per cent. There is also uncertainty in the third step of the calibration, the calibration of the BCR rabbit thromboplastin against the IRP, and this will increase the total CV of the calibration to 10.5 per cent. The uncertainty in an INR is also dependent on the variability of points about the calibration line. Again the magnitude of the standard deviation about the orthogonal regression line for a calibration of a production lot of rabbit thromboplastin against the IRP is not known. Calibration of the BCR rabbit thromboplastin against the IRP would suggest a figure of not less than 0.030.

These estimates of the precision of a calibration of a production lot against the IRP and the standard deviation about the orthogonal regression line can be used to estimate the uncertainty in an INR derived from that calibration. To simplify the calculation it will also be assumed that the production lot and house standard have the same sensitivity as the BCR rabbit thromboplastin. Hence the slope of the calibration lines of the house standard against the BCR rabbit thromboplastin and a production lot against the house standard are both 1.0. The slope of the calibration line of the BCR rabbit thromboplastin against the IRP was found to be 1.413 in the BCR study which by assumption is also the slope of the calibration line of the production lot against the IRP. Let R_{PL} be a patient's prothrombin ratio with a production lot, b and s(b) the slope and standard error of the calibration line of the production lot against the IRP, and s the standard deviation about the orthogonal regression line. Then the standard error of the logarithm of the INR corresponding to the ratio R_{PL}, s(log INR), is approximated by

$$s(\log \text{INR}) = \left[(s(b) \log R_{PL})^2 + (1 + b^2) s^2 \right]^{\frac{1}{2}} \qquad \text{(Equation 4)}$$

The upper and lower limits of a 95% confidence interval for the INR are given by

$$R_{PL}^b \cdot 10^{-1.96 s(\log \text{INR})} \quad \text{and} \quad R_{PL}^b \cdot 10^{1.96 s(\log \text{INR})}$$

It has already been demonstrated that the variability in b expressed as a CV is of the order of 10.5%. Thus s(b) is given by b·(10.5/100) and s is taken to be 0.030. With these assumptions an interval of 2.47-4.96 is calculated for an INR estimated at 3.5, the mid-point of the therapeutic range 2.0-5. This is a wide interval and it is clear that some patients whose INR is well within the therapeutic range could actually be underdosed or overdosed. Nevertheless this is probably the worst case likely to occur in practice and the position could be considerably improved if manufacturers obtained independent estimates of the calibration of the house standard against the BCR rabbit thromboplastin.

For conversion of prothrombin ratios a further component should be included in the standard error of prediction to account for the variation in the mean normal prothrombin time. This term is of less importance as it is given by s^2/n, where s^2 is the average variation of observations about the calibration line and n the number of normals used to calculate the prothrombin ratio. It should also be noted that no allowance has been made for the fact that the calibration line is to be used repeatedly. It is well known (11) that any errors in the calibration line are perpetuated in all the determinations for which it is used. Consequently the proportion of confidence intervals failing to include the true value will be appreciably larger than the stated significance level. An adjustment can be made to ensure that the requisite proportion of confidence intervals determined using the same calibration line will bracket their true values.

4. CLINICAL APPLICABILITY

Loeliger and Lewis (12) state that the use of BCR reference materials and the adoption of INRs will greatly facilitate the application of common and well defined therapeutic ranges, independent of the type of thromboplastin used. They have proposed ranges expressed as INRs and as ratios with the BCR reference materials for various clinical conditions for both in-patients and out-patients. However, the protocol of the BCR study specifies that patients used for calibration should have recovered their general health (preferably out-patients) and have been stabilised on anticoagulation for at least six weeks. The theory underlying anticoagulation would suggest there is no reason to assume that certified values obtained using such patients can be used to calculate INRs for patients in the early stages of therapy. Coumarin-type anticoagulants induce a combined depression of the coagulation Factors II, VII, IX, and X with Factor VII being reduced first and Factor II more slowly. Individual thromboplastin reagents vary considerably in their sensitivity to the Factors II, VII and X and it might be anticipated that different calibration results would be achieved for patients in the early stages.

Table 2. The standard deviations about the calibration line for long-term and short-term patients.

| | Calibration | | |
	BCT/253 vs Simplastin	BCT/253 vs RBT/79	Simplastin vs RBT/79
long-term	0.021	0.017	0.021
short-term	0.031	0.019	0.028

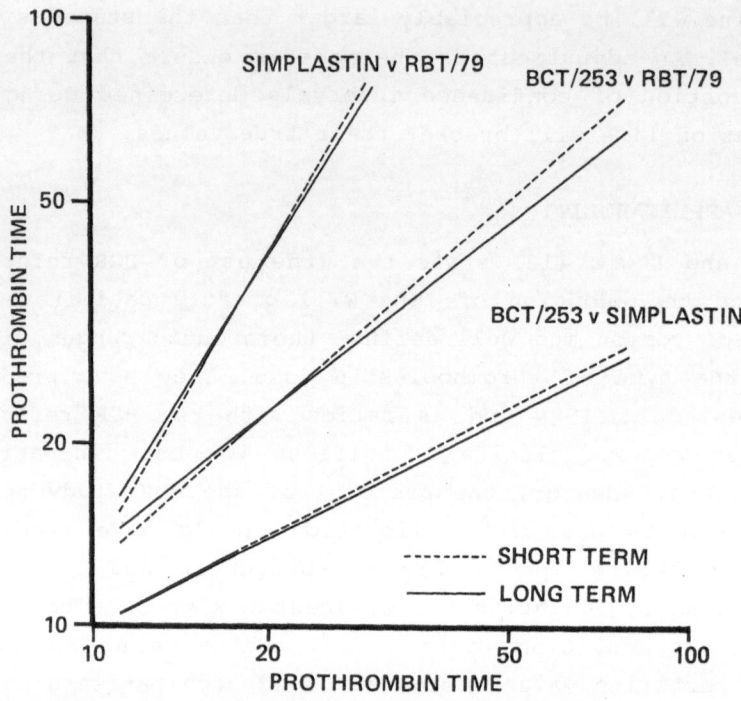

FIGURE 5. Calibration lines are shown for long- and short-term coumarin-treated patients. In each case the prothrombin times obtained with the first mentioned thromboplastin are on the x-axis.

To investigate this hypothesis, the commercial rabbit tissue extract Simplastin has been calibrated against two reference thromboplastins, the proposed IRP (BCT/253) and the BCR rabbit thromboplastin (RBT/79), in two separate exercises. The first calibration excercise included only long-term stabilised patients as specified in the BCR-protocol. The second set of calibrations were performed on patients who had undergone less than three weeks of coumarin therapy. The results of these calibration exercises are shown in Figure 5 and Table 2. The calibration lines for short-term and long-term coumarin-treated patients are shown in Fig. 5. It can be seen that for each of the three calibrations there is little difference between the calibration lines. The principal difference between the two series of calibrations was found in the standard deviations about the calibration line. They are given in Table 2 where it can be seen that the variation about the calibration line is greater for short-term patients. In other words the procedure is less dependable in non-stabilized patients. The effect was much more marked for those patients seen during the first five days of therapy although the numbers were too few to draw firm conclusions.

5. CHOICE OF CALIBRATION SEQUENCE

The new calibration scheme is hierarchical; starting with the WHO primary reference thromboplastin, the IRP, calibration proceeds through secondary reference preparations and production lots of manufacturers down to the prothrombin time test on an individual patient. There are three BCR reference thromboplastins available to manufacturers against which they may calibrate their products. The BCR calibration protocol recommends that they use the reference of the same species because it is felt that for this calibration the variation of prothrombin times about the line is the least. In the BCR study this was the case for two of the three BCR reference materials when calibrated against their WHO counterparts. However, re-analysis of the BCR data has shown that the principal factor influencing the variability of prothrombin times about the line is not the species effect i.e. whether of human or animal origin, but whether the "like-to-like" relationship related to the composition of the reagent i.e. whether it is the usual Quick test reagent or manufactured with added plasma.

Table 3. Characteristics of WHO and BCR thromboplastin reference materials.

	67/40	68/434	70/178	BCT/099	OBT/79	RBT/79
brain tissue type	human	bovine	rabbit	human	bovine	rabbit
manufacture	combined	combined	plain	plain	combined	plain

Table 3 characterises the WHO and BCR reference preparations in terms of the brain tissue from which they were prepared and whether they were manufactured with added fibrinogen and coagulation Factor V. The terms combined and plain are used to denote those preparations manufactured with and without added fibrinogen and coagulation Factor V, respectively. Figures 6, 7, 8 show 95% confidence intervals for ratios with each of the three WHO reference thromboplastins (human, bovine and rabbit) corresponding to prothrombin ratios with the other thromboplastin included in the study. These predicted ratios are the ratios on the reference material scale which correspond to the mean ratio of patients obtained with the other thromboplastins. In each case it can be seen that the best calibration, as measured by the width of the intervals, is obtained when thromboplastins mutually similar in terms of composition are calibrated against each other. In addition to this composition effect there is a less important secondary species effect.

For the IRP, 67/40, which is a human combined reagent the best calibration is against the bovine combined reagents. However, amongst the plain reagents, the best calibration is against the BCR human brain reagent BCT/099. The bovine WHO reference preparation, a combined reagent, calibrates best against the BCR bovine thromboplastin. In the case of 70/178 a plain, rabbit reagent, the best calibration is achieved against the BCR human and rabbit thromboplastins, both plain reagents. The calibration against the BCR rabbit thromboplastin is only marginally better than against the BCR human thromboplastin and would make little practical difference. The Quick prothrombin time test is the procedure used in the hospitals of most countries for anticoagulant control (13). This result strengthens the case put forward by Ingram (14) for the replacement of the WHO IRP which is a combined reagent by the proposed second IRP which is a human brain Quick test (plain) reagent.

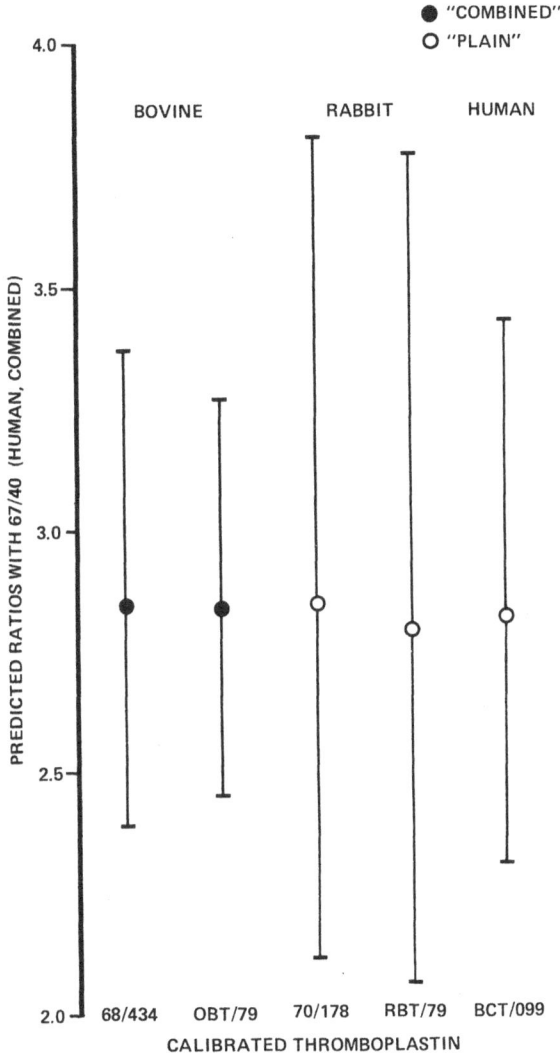

FIGURE 6. Approximate 95% confidence intervals for predicted ratios with the WHO reference thromboplastin human. Calibration relationships have been used to predict the mean prothrombin ratio with the reference thromboplastin from the mean pro-thrombin ratio of each thromboplastin included in the study.

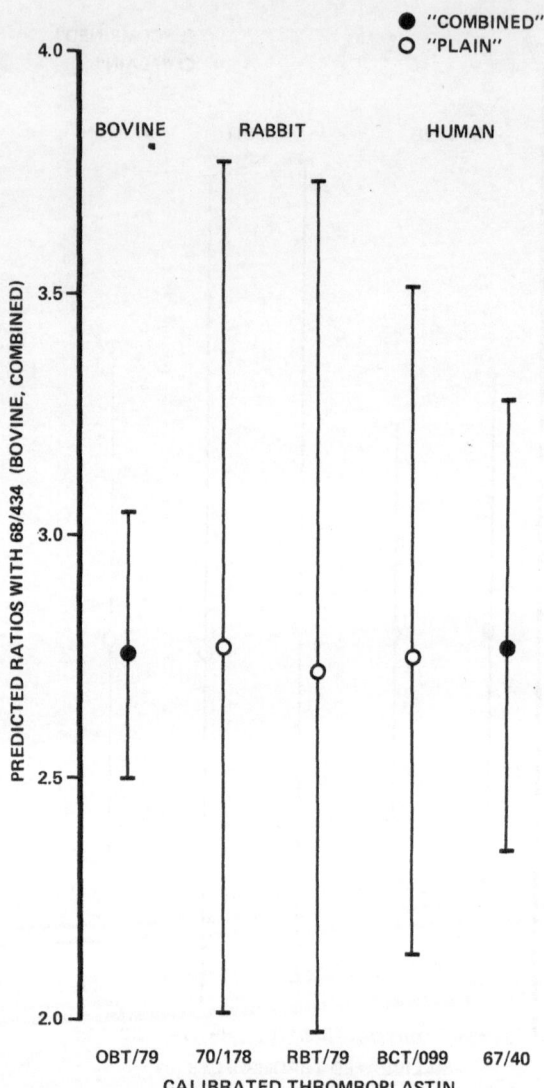

FIGURE 7. Approximate 95% confidence intervals for predicted ratios with the WHO reference thromboplastin bovine. Calibration relationships have been used to predict the mean prothrombin ratio with the reference thromboplastin from the mean prothrombin ratio of each thromboplastin included in the study.

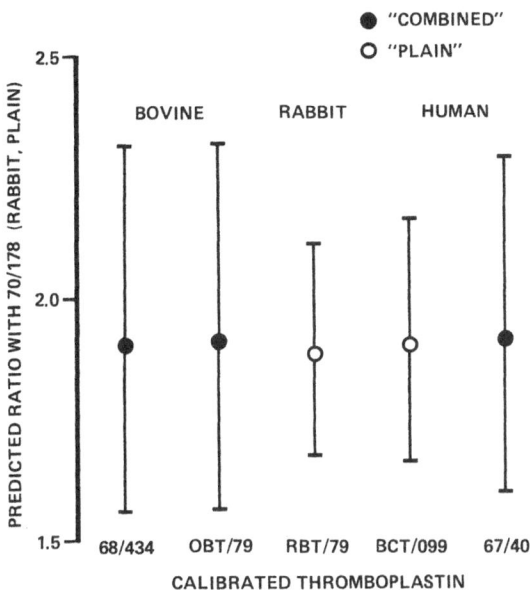

FIGURE 8. Approximate 95% confidence intervals for predicted ratios with the WHO reference thromboplastin rabbit. Calibration relationships have been used to predict the mean prothrombin ratio with the reference thromboplastin from the mean prothrombin ratio of each thromboplastin included in the study.

REFERENCES

1. Loeliger EA, Van den Besselaar AMHP, Hermans J, Van der Velde EA. Certification of three reference materials for thromboplastins. BCR information, Commission of the European Communities, Brussels 1981.
2. Poller L. The British comparative thromboplastin: The use of the national thromboplastin reagent for uniformity of laboratory control of oral anticoagulants and expression of results. Association of Clinical Pathologists. 1970; Broadsheet No. 71.

3. WHO Expert Committee on Biological Standardization. 28th Report. WHO technical Report Series 610. World Health Organization, Geneva 1977: pp. 14-15 and 45-51.

4. WHO Expert Committee on Biological Standardization. 31st Report. WHO Technical Report Series 658. World Health Organization, Geneva 1981: pp. 185-215.

5. Biggs R, Denson KWE. Standardization of the one-stage prothrombin time for the control of anticoagulant therapy. Br Med J 1967; 1:84-88.

6. Kirkwood TBL. Calibration of reference thromboplastins and standardization of the prothrombin time ratio. Thromb Haemostas (Stuttgart) 1983; 49:238-244.

7. Thomson JM, Stevenson KJ, Tomenson JA. Report on proposed second WHO international reference thromboplastin, human, plain, to replace the WHO international reference preparation, human, combined. Submitted to WHO. 1983.

8. Tomenson JA, Thomson JM, Poller L. The British system of oral anticoagulant control and its relation with the WHO system: calibration of the proposed second WHO international reference thromboplastin (BCT/253). This volume, chapter 9.

9. Van den Besselaar AMHP, Van der Velde EA. The Manufacturers' Calibration Study. This volume, chapter 7.

10. Hermans J, Van den Besselaar AMHP den, Loeliger EA, Van der Velde EA. A collaborative calibration study of reference materials for thromboplastins. Thromb Haemostas 1983;

11. Mandel J. The statistical analysis of experimental data. John Wiley and Sons, New York 1964.

12. Loeliger EA, Lewis SM. Progress in laboratory control of oral anticoagulants. Lancet 1982; II, 318-320.

13. Lam-Po Tang PRLC, Poller L. Oral anticoagulant therapy and its control: An International Survey. Thrombosis et Diathes Haemorrh (Stuttg) 1975; 34:419-425.

14. Ingram GIC. The stability of the WHO reference thromboplastin NIBS&C 67/40. Thromb Haemostas (Stuttgart) 1979;42: 1135-1140.

APPENDIX

Technical note concerning the test of the assumption that the mean logarithms of the prothrombin times of normals lie on the orthogonal regression line through patients' plasmas.

An approximate test was used to examine the assumption that the mean logarithms of the prothrombin times of normals are found on the orthogonal regression line derived using patients' plasma. The test is based on that of Welch (1947) used for comparisons of means involving two variances which must be separately estimated. The test statistic is derived from the residual deviation of the mean logarithms of the prothrombin times of normals.

Let $\bar{x}_N$, $\bar{y}_N$ be the mean logarithms of the prothrombin times of normals and a, b the intercept and slope of the orthogonal regression line calculated using only the results of patients. If the assumption is correct, then

$$d = \bar{y}_N - a - b\bar{x}_N \tag{1}$$

has zero mean.

Write b as $\beta + \varepsilon_b$, $\bar{x}_N$ as $\mu_N + \varepsilon_N$ where β, μ_N are the true underlying values and ε_b, ε_N the random components. Then $b\bar{x}_N$ may be written as

$$\beta\bar{x}_N + \mu_N\varepsilon_b + \varepsilon_b\varepsilon_N \tag{2}$$

The final term of (2) may be ignored because it is much smaller in magnitude than the other terms in the expression.

Thus approximately d can be regarded as the sum of two random components.

$$\bar{y}_N - \beta\bar{x}_N \tag{3}$$

$$-a - b\mu_N \tag{4}$$

and a fixed term $\beta\mu_N$.

If n_N is the number of normals, then an estimate of the variance of (3) based on $n_N - 1$ degrees of freedom is given by

$$s_1^2 = (s_y^2 - 2brs_xs_y + b^2s_x^2)/n_N,$$ (5)

where S_x, S_y are the standard deviations of the logarithms of prothrombin times for normals and r their correlation.

If n_p is the number of patient plasmas, an estimate of the variance of (4) based on $n_p - 2$ degrees of freedom is

$$s_2^2 = s_a^2 + \bar{x}_N^2 s_b^2 + 2\bar{x}_N r_{ab} s_a s_b$$ (6)

where S_a, S_b and r_{ab} are estimates of the standard error of a and b and the correlation of a and b given by Patefield (1977).

The test of Welch can be used by treating (3), (4) as normal variates with separately estimated variances.

The test statistic is

$$v = \frac{d}{[s_1^2 + s_2^2]^{\frac{1}{2}}}$$

and significance levels for the test which depend on the degrees of freedom of s_1^2, s_2^2, and the ratio $s_1^2 : s_2^2$ have been tabulated (Biometrika Tables, Vol I, Table II). The test is approximate, particularly the estimate s_2^2 which utilises an asymptotic covariance matrix, and a conservative significance level should be used.

REFERENCES

Patefield WM. On the information matrix in the linear functional relationship problem. Applied Statistics 1977; 26:69-70.
Pearson ES, Hartley HO (eds) Biometrika Tables for Statisticians. London. Biometrika Trust, 1976.
Welch BL. The generalisation of 'Students' problem when several different population variances are involved. Biometrika 1947; 34:28.

Chapter 6:   CRITICAL REMARKS FROM A CLINICIAN'S POINT OF VIEW

E.A. LOELIGER

With respect to the clinical impact of thromboplastin calibration, the key question is: "What implications does the use of
different thromboplastins and their conversion into each other
terms by means of thromboplastin calibration. have for dosage
regulation in the individual patient?". For the answer to this
question consideration of at least three variables is of importance: first, the parameters of the line of correlation used to
convert a prothrombin time found with one thromboplastin into the
terms of that of the other thromboplastin. Second, the thromboplastin specific deviation of the prothrombin time of an individual patient from the correlation line; and third, the patient
specific fluctuation of successive prothrombin times during the
period of his treatment.

Table 1 Coefficient of variation of slope (b) and intercept (I) for
the BCR reference thromboplastins

	$\frac{SD\ b}{b} \times 100$	$\frac{SEM\ b}{b} \times 100$	$\frac{SD\ I}{I} \times 100$	$\frac{SEM\ I}{I} \times 100$
BCT/099	3.8	1.4	8.1	3.0
OBT/79	4.0	1.5	5.0	1.9
RBT/79	6.8	2.6	13.7	5.2

I = prothrombin time/sec for the IRP (67/40) in the middle of the
therapeutic range (I=62.4, corresponding to 3.5 INR)
SEM = Standard Error of the Mean (for 7 European laboratories)

Table 1 summarizes the magnitude of the inaccuracy of the
slopes and intercepts (in the middle of the therapeutic range) of
the lines of the three certified BCR materials. At the left-hand

side the standard deviations (SD) and standard errors of the means (SEM) are presented for the slopes of the line, and at the right-hand side SD and SEM for the intercepts in the therapeutic range. The inaccuracy with which a single laboratory of a thromboplastin manufacturer assesses the slope of the relationship for its house standard is not known. Its magnitude can, however, be deduced by analogy from the BCR study (1) and the Manchester calibration study (2). In terms of coefficient of variation (CV), the magnitude approximates 5 per cent, the limit set by WHO recommendations for the precision with which the ISI of a house standard thromboplastin should be assessed by individual laboratories (in the BCR study and the Manchester study, the interlaboratory variations for the ISIs were 3.8-6.8 and 5%, respectively). In order not to surpass the 5 per cent limits, we recommend that house standard calibration be performed with carefully collected samples of patients on stable oral anticoagulation, and - for rabbit thromboplastins plain - preferably by two independent laboratories. It is good to know, that the third and last step in the hierarchy of thromboplastin calibration, namely that of the calibration of successive batches of one production series does not, in our experience, create problems. Its inaccuracy is easily kept within a CV of 2.5 % (3). Therefore, the cumulated inaccuracy of the slope (ISI) can be kept within the limits defined by a CV of 5-6 %.

The second variable in the estimation of an INR is the magnitude of the thromboplastin specific deviation of the prothrombin time as measured in an individual patient sample. For expert laboratories we know that if different types of thromboplastin and different techniques are compared, the coefficient of variation quantifying this effect amounts, for prothrombin times around the therapeutic target, up to 8%. However, for like procedures or like tissue types of thromboplastin it amounts to not more than 4-5%.

Thirdly, the fluctuation of patient specific prothrombin times as measured over time of treatment amounts, for a thromboplastin with an ISI approximating 1, such as is used in our thrombosis centre, to a value between 10 and 15% (CV). In relation to this

variation, the 5-6% CV of the ISI inaccuracy pales into insignificance.

The important question now is whether prothrombin time monitoring in the individual patient in a given centre indeed is
thromboplastin independent as it would seem to be from the
aforementioned reasoning. To investigate this point, a prospective double-blind study was launched some years ago at the Leiden
Thrombosis Centre in more than 800 patients on stable oral
anticoagulation (4). The patients were randomly allocated to
three groups, one continuing to be monitored with Thrombotest,
and in the two others Thrombotest was replaced by either British
Comparative Thromboplastin or Simplastin Automated, but dosage
regulation in both occurring with Thrombotest equivalents calcu-

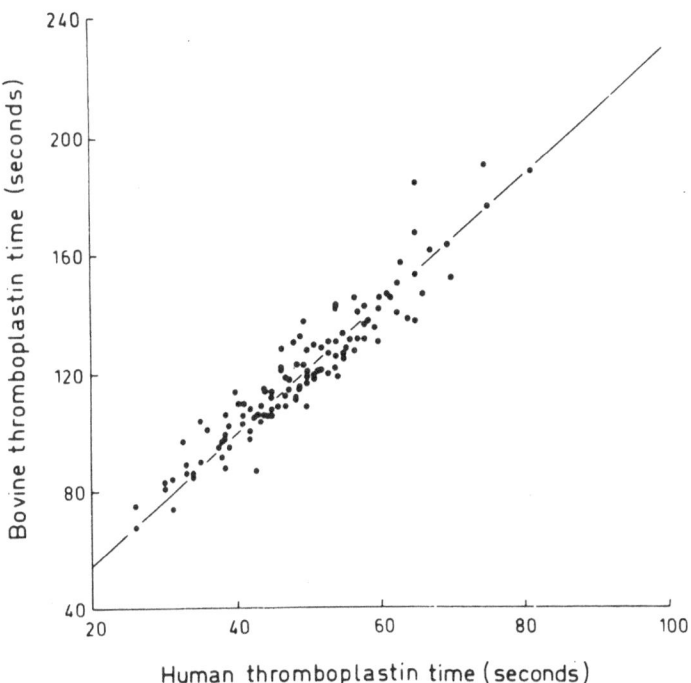

FIGURE 1. Correlation between prothrombin times (PTs) assessed
with bovine thromboplastin (BT) and human thromboplastin (HT) for
125 patients. The line is defined by the calibration equation
BT = 12.44 + 2.19HT. (Reproduced with permission from the Am J
Clin Pathol 1981; 75: 297-303.)

112

lated from the calibration relationship as empirically established by thromboplastin calibration (Figs. 1-4). In spite of the
considerable scattering of the individual prothrombin times
around the calibration line for BCT as well as for Simplastin
Automated it became clear within 8 months from the start of the
trial, that prothrombin times obtained with BCT and with Simplastin Automated were just as safe for patient monitoring as with
Thrombotest itself.

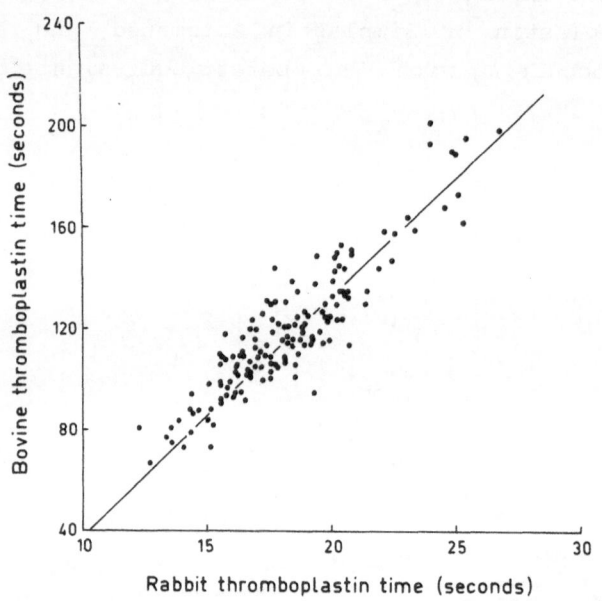

FIGURE 2. Correlation between prothrombin times (PTs) assessed
with bovine thromboplastin (BT) and rabbit thromboplastin (RT)
for 169 patients. The line is defined by the calibration equation
BT = -52.35 + 9.38RT. (Reproduced with permission from the Am J
Clin Pathol 1981; 75: 297-303.)

To demonstrate the relative insignificance of the calibration
inaccuracy in the clinical practice of dosage regulation even
more tangibly for today's discussion, I translated, for a sample
representative for the whole study, the prothrombin times measur-

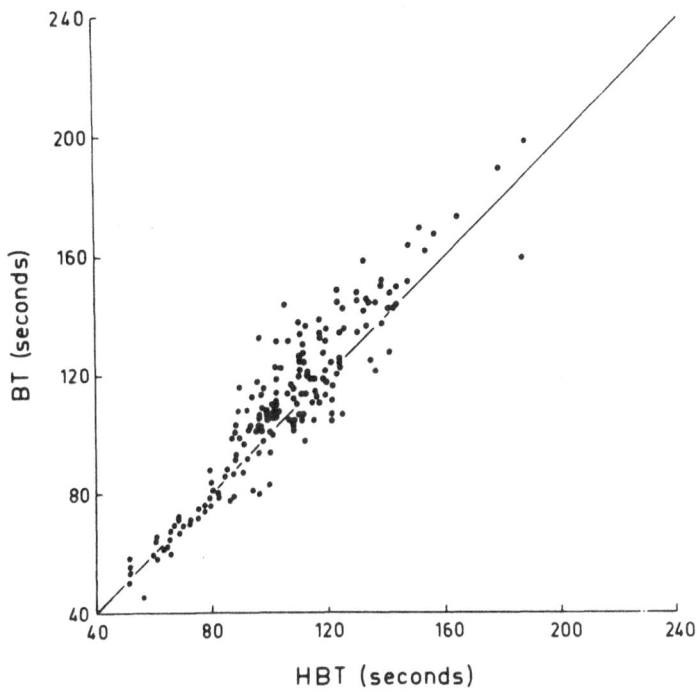

FIGURE 3. Relationship between prothrombin times (PTs) measured with bovine thromboplastin (BT) and calculated PTs (HBT, i.e., PTs measured with human thromboplastin and converted into terms of bovine thromboplastin). The conversion was based on the calibration equation BT = 12.44 + 2.19HT. (Reproduced with permission from the Am J Clin Pathol 1981; 75: 297-303.)

Table 2

	ISI	mean normal prothrombin time
BOVINE (Thrombotest)	1.02	39 sec (Lode coagu-lometer)
HUMAN (BCT, liquid)	1.0	15 sec (tilt-tube technique)
RABBIT (Simplastin Automated)	1.9	10 sec (Sherwood coagulyzer)

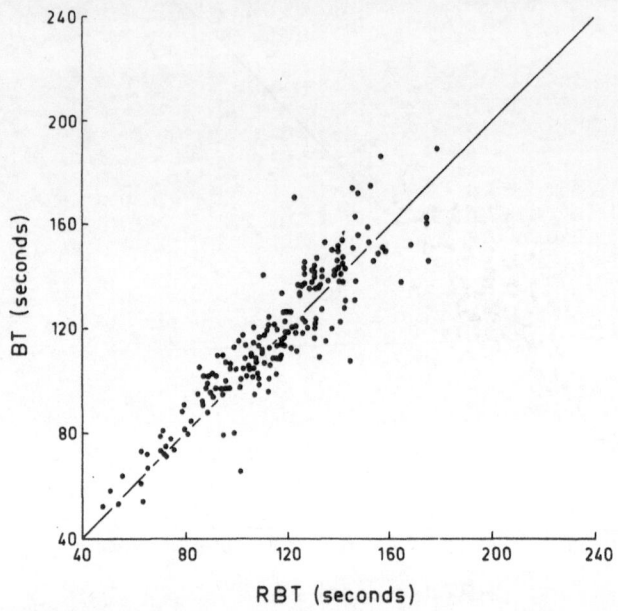

FIGURE 4. Relationship between prothrombin times (PTs) measured with bovine thromboplastin (BT) and calculated PTs (RBT, i.e., PTs measured with rabbit thromboplastin and converted into terms of bovine thromboplastin). The conversion was based on the calibration equation $BT = -52.35 + 9.38RT$. (Reproduced with permission from the Am J Clin Pathol 1981; 75: 297-303.)

ed in the patients of the three study groups into International Normalized Ratios (INRs), using fixed ISI values and fixed mean normal PTs for all three thromboplastins (Table 2), for the whole eight-month period of observation. For Thrombotest and Simplastin Automated, only one batch was used throughout the study. The between thromboplastin CV of the INRs calculated with the values shown in Table 2 approximated 8% for both the pair BCT/ Thrombotest and the pair Simplastin Automated/Thrombotest. Table 3 shows the means of the INRs as calculated for the three groups on eight randomly chosen observation days of the study. As expected for well-calibrated thromboplastins, the differences between the

Table 3 Mean INR equivalents as calculated for prothrombin times
obtained on eight different days in the three groups of
patients studied by Boekhout-Mussert et al. (Amer J Clin
Path 1981; 75: 297-303)

date in 1977	GROUP I bov only		GROUP II hum bov			GROUP III rab bov		
04.02	3.4	(17)	3.4	3.3	(14)	3.0	3.2	(12)
11.02	3.2	(18)	3.3	3.2	(16)	3.6	3.6	(18)
23.03	3.0	(16)	3.6	3.4	(14)	3.4	3.4	(17)
20.04	3.1	(13)	3.0	3.1	(16)	3.3	3.3	(15)
25.05	3.0	(13)	3.3	3.3	(19)	3.1	3.2	(12)
15.06	3.3	(16)	3.4	3.2	(10)	3.4	3.3	(14)
12.07	3.6	(13)	3.3	3.3	(17)	3.4	3.3	(14)
12.08	3.3	(8)	4.1	3.9	(6)	3.6	3.7	(11)
mean of 8 days	3.25	(114)	3.40	3.35	(112)	3.35	3.35	(113)

numbers of patients are indicated between brackets.

means per pair per day were small, amounting to a CV of not more
than 2.5 per cent.

Please note too the magnitude of the mean intensity of anticoagulation achieved, which was about 3.3 INR. More than 80 per
cent of the INRs remained within the range of 2.5-5.

In sum: out-patient monitoring with calibrated thromboplastins of different tissue types and with different assay techniques was feasible and clinically safe in a prospective double-
blind randomized trial. Calibration inaccuracy plays only a minor
role in the inter-thromboplastin variation. Influences of individual nature of the patients are more pronounced.

REFERENCES

1. Loeliger EA, Van den Besselaar AMHP, Hermans J, Van der Velde
    EA. Certification of three reference materials for throm-
    boplastins; BCR CRM no. 147, 148, 149. BCR information.
    Commission of the European Communities, 200 rue de la Loi,
    1049 Brussels, Belgium. 1981.

2. Thomson JM, Stevenson KJ, Tomenson JA. Report on proposed second WHO international reference thromboplastin. Submitted to WHO, 1983.
3. Loeliger EA, Van der Hoeff-van Halem R, Van Halem-Visser LP. Thromboplastin calibration. Experience of the Dutch Reference Laboratory for Anticoagulant Control. Thromb Haemostas 1978; 40: 272-287.
4. Boekhout-Mussert MJ, Van der Kolk-Schaap PJ, Hermans J, Loeliger EA. Prospective double-blind clinical trial of bovine, human, and rabbit thromboplastins in monitoring long-term oral anticoagulation. Am J Clin Path 1981; 75: 297-303.

DISCUSSION

CHAIRMEN: K.W.E. DENSON
          H.R. GRALNICK

POLLER: We have now an agreed international method (internatio-
        nal normalised ratios - INR) for quantifying the dif-
        ferences between reagents on which in the past a precise
        figure could not be put, but were known to be sub-
        stantial.
        I wish to refer to a study published in 1982 in the New
        England Journal of Medicine by the McMaster group (1) to
        exemplify this point. The figure shows the value of the
        INR approach in quantitating the differences between
        thromboplastins. The trial was instituted at the sugges-
        tion of the Europeans to try to convince their North
        American colleagues that their intensity of anticoagula-
        tion was too great and that the incidence of haemorrhage
        could be reduced by applying the type of therapeutic
        range customarily used in the UK and The Netherlands.
        The McMaster group undertook a randomised prospective
        trial with two methods of Quick test control, i.e.
        Manchester Reagent (ISI 0.99) used in over 90% of UK
        hospitals, and Simplastin. The latter is one of the most
        popular and widely used commercial reagents. They aimed
        at a prothrombin ratio 2.0 on both scales. The results
        of this trial were that protection against re-thrombosis
        in patients with recent venous thrombosis was equal with
        the two systems, but that the incidence of haemorrhage
        was much reduced by the more conservative dosage regimen
        using the Manchester Reagent control.
        A ratio of 2.0 on the Simplastin scale is in fact
        equivalent to 57 seconds with the Manchester Reagent,

118

according to the INR scale. A ratio of 2.0 with Simplastin would be equated on the INR scale to 4.5. There is
in fact a considerable scatter of results in the
McMaster trial which gave 57 seconds with MCR on the
same plasma samples. At one end of the scale the clinician will be underdosing or bound to increase the
patient's dose, whereas the other extreme of results
equivalent to MCR with Simplastin are in the bleeding
zone! The circles and triangles indicate bleeding
episodes which occurred in the study.

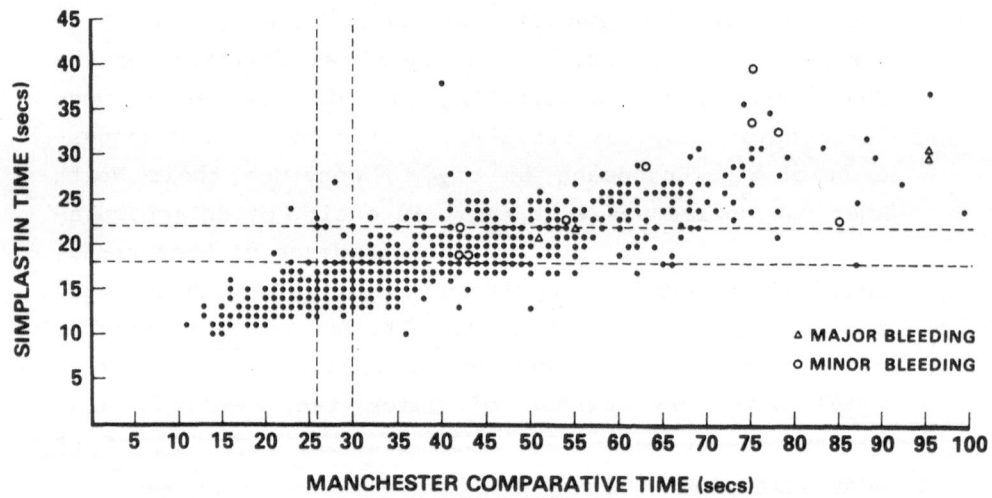

FIGURE: Relation between the Simplastin times and the Manchester
Comparative times determined in aliquots of the same plasma
samples from all patients over the three-month course of therapy. Many points represent multiple overlapping prothrombin-time
results. The prothrombin-time responses at the time of bleeding
are also indicated for each patient who had major and minor
bleeding complications. All 13 who bled did so when the Manchester Comparative time was prolonged to more than three times that
of the control, whereas 12 of the 13 patients bled when the
Simplastin time was less than three times that of the control.
The dotted lines indicate the therapeutic ranges, set before the
study began. (reprinted by permission of The New England Journal
of Medicine 1982; 307: 1676-1681).

In other words, patients bled at a level which should be safe on the INR scale. The answer is not to denigrate the INR principle but to emphasise two points. These were all short-term patients within the first three months of treatment and results of the correlations between reagents are relatively poor at this stage.

Secondly, in the early days of therapy the active forms of vitamin K-dependent clotting factors II, VII, IX and X disappear at varying rates from the circulation. Simplastin is relatively insensitive to factor VII as is the case with many commercial reagents. The INR system however gives the manufacturers a target of sensitivity which they have not had before. They can see if they can improve the correlation of their reagents with the International Reference Preparation. Until that is done, INRs in the early days of treatment will be relatively meaningless and perhaps dangerous in terms of patient therapy. The INR principle (which quantifies precisely the difference between these thromboplastins in general terms but not precisely in terms of an individual patient's results) gives the manufacturers a target. They may ultimately evolve a common type of thromboplastin measuring the vitamin K-dependent factors to a similar extent. That would be the optimum solution.

LOELIGER: I think that in the early stages many of the samples were under the influence not only of coumarin but also of heparin. Simplastin is heavily heparin-sensitive whereas the Manchester Reagent is insensitive to even therapeutic doses of heparin. This may explain at least part of the enormous scatter.

POLLER: Some patients, throughout their period of therapy, gave mean prothrombin time values which were within the normal range or minimally prolonged on the Simplastin scale even though parallel tests were therapeutic with Manchester Reagent. They were proven to be protected clinically by the trial. This type of result occurred not just in the early days of treatment but throughout the course of therapy and therefore could not be a heparin effect.

TOMENSON: Professor Loeliger has referred to errors which in many instances were half the size of those mentioned by myself. This is because he has used coefficients of variation to quantify standard error, whereas I have taken the limits of a 95% confidence interval. However, Professor Loeliger's error limits only include the true value 70% of the time and do not fully reflect the error involved.

COLINET: I would like to know what you mean by 95% confidence interval.

TOMENSON: I think you were referring to the taking of a slope estimate from one laboratory and applying that result to all laboratories. In this case an approximate 95% confidence interval can be seen as being twice the coefficient of between-laboratory variation that Professor Loeliger has quoted.

COLINET: There is a confusion between the confidence interval and tolerance interval. A confidence interval refers only to the mean, and a tolerance interval would refer to the population of results. That is why I think you had a disagreement when you quoted the values stated in the BCR-report and the individual values.

SHINTON: Can any of the speakers of this morning offer an explanation as to why there is a difference in the linear relationship between the lower levels with normals compared with the high levels that you are getting with the patients on anticoagulants when comparing two thromboplastins?

KIRKWOOD: Although those differences in slope are statistically significant, I think it is important to bear in mind that in the case of the normals you are putting a line through a very tight cluster of points. There is no obvious statistical reason why this should be important, but there may well be a biochemical reason.

SPAETHE: I think it is a question of PIVKA. When you compare PIVKA-insensitive and PIVKA-sensitive thromboplastins, you find a linear relationship with normals and liver patients, but not with anticoagulated patients.

LOELIGER: Prof. Hemker would probably add that one thromboplastin is much more sensitive to PIVKA X (in the example it was Thrombotest) than the other thromboplastin.

DENSON: I have two problems that I would like the statisticians to answer. The first one relates to the range of ISIs that were obtained in the BCR-study. These range from 1.3 to 1.59. It worries me a little because these are fractional powers as well but it means in fact that if you had chosen laboratory 3 to do the entire study (I know you take a mean of all ten laboratories), but had you used the samples in laboratory 3, you would have got a very different result to laboratory 8. I think this is due to the degree of anticoagulation. If we take laboratory 8 and calculate an INR, we get an INR of 4.17 with an X-value of 3, and 5.74 with the same X-value for laboratory 3. I think this may well be due to PIVKA but that is not the whole story. It could be due to the dilution effects of the different thromboplastins, but there are other variables.

KIRKWOOD: The answer I would make is a rather general one. It is based on experience with attempts to introduce biological standardization in a number of different areas of coagulation. No standardization programme is going to produce exact agreement between different laboratories. For example, if you take coagulation factor assays, in collaborative studies where you send out identical lyophilized preparations and ask each laboratory to assay one preparation against another, then you find that among, say, ten laboratories you can have as much as a two-fold difference in potency ratio between the top and the bottom of the range.

DENSON: This is not random error, but systematic error.

KIRKWOOD: It is a fact of life in biological standardization that when you do a multi-center collaborative study you will get systematic differences between centers. The aim it to try to identify the causes of those differences and to introduce further standardization, so as to minimize differences in subsequent attempts.
Looking at the numbers you have on the slide, if the worst discrepancy is between laboratory 8 and laboratory 3, and the difference is between an INR of 4.17 and 5.74, then by comparison with other areas of standardization, this is a really excellent position. One has to accept that there are going to be factors that are not allowed for in the standardization system, which is trying to reduce a lot of variation into a simple relationship. It is certainly not ideal, but I think it is really very good.

DENSON: I am not questioning its goodness. It is a very nice study. It achieved what it set out to do. But there is a real difference, i.e. the ISI that we put on a thromboplastin is clearly dependent on the degree of anticoagulation within that laboratory.

LOELIGER: Dr. Denson, you are always skillful in identifying the exceptions. You probably have seen that the 1.59 value is an outlier in the series of 10. I know this laboratory very well and I suppose that there was a systematic exception, not due to general influences but due to human influences. On repetition, we find a slope which is no longer far different from the slopes of the 9 other laboratories. This mitigates it a little. You have chosen the example which is the most flagrant example of disagreement.

DENSON: I think the other point was, that laboratory 2 and laboratory 3 also had extremes, but laboratory 3 had about twice the degree of anticoagulation in terms of ratios.

DOMBROSE: I would like to address a couple of points to dr. Van der Velde with regard to the orthogonal regression. It seems to me that there is some systematic bias in the data with regard to the reagents that are PIVKA-sensitive. If this is true, and the orthogonal regression is the regression we should be using, would you tell us of the effect of non-homogeneity of variance in the data and how any systematic bias or statistically inconsistent relationships can affect the orthogonal regression?

VAN DER VELDE: It is for mathematical reasons that we have to specify the ratio of the variances or more specially to assume equality of the variances. As soon as one has information that this cannot be justified, the calculation should be modified. In that case simple modifications of the equations are needed. Algebraically speaking, one first multiplies the data with a constant, to make the error variance in one direction equal to that in the other direction. Then one proceeds by orthogonal regression. The name "orthogonal regression" stems from the situation where the variances are equal. In statistical textbooks on functional relationships, the authors don't refer to orthogonality but they give equations which include the ratio of variances.

DENSON: I think there is one important point which relates to the BCR study. The statisticians analyzed the results and they produced sensitivity indices for each laboratory and they also produced calibration constants based on the mean values ("Biggs-Denson") line. The correlation coefficient for the calibration constants against the sensitivity indices was 0.97. In other words, there is absolutely no difference between using the "mean values line" and using log PT regression.

LOELIGER: There is indeed little clinically important difference as long as you stick to 1.5 to 5 (INR). Many of our colleagues abroad tend to anticoagulate between 3 and 10 INR and then you will find less agreement.

DENSON: I agree with that, but if you go outside this range, the ISI means nothing. I am convinced that the ISI is dependent ultimately on the degree of anticoagulation of the samples.

KIRKWOOD: The difference is not in the actual numbers that emerge but in the way the calibration is done. In the remarks I made earlier, I indicated what the nature of the difference was. One general comment needs to be made, and that is that in the presentation of the new calibration model and in the discussion of orthogonal regression, the impression may be received that the new calibration system is intrinsically more complicated that the system it replaces. This is not true. If you were to do the same sort of statistical appraisal with the ratio plot, you would also require orthogonal regression. The requirement for orthogonal regression is simply a consequence of the fact that there is variation on both axes. Furthermore, although the formulae for the standard deviation and the formulae for testing the validity of the model in the log-seconds plot seem more complex than anything that was published in the original

WHO requirements, this is just a reflection of the fact that no indication was given previously as to how you would actually analyse the calibration statistically. If you were to try to do that with the earlier calibration system, you would have much more complex formulae, because you would be dealing with a model which was not amenable to any kind of conventional statistical analysis. The reason for this is that, as I stated previously, you would be trying to analyse ratios where the denominator of the ratio (the mean normal prothrombin time) disappears in the plot, but nevertheless has to be taken into account in the statistical analysis. To handle the equations for that case would be a nightmare.

REFERENCE

1. Hull R, Hirsh J, Jay R, Carter C, England C, Gent M, Turpie AGG, McLoughlin D, Dodd P, Thomas M, Raskob G, Ockleford P. Different intensities of oral anticoagulation therapy in the treatment of proximal-vein thrombosis. N Engl J Med 1982; 307: 1676-1681.

Chapter 7:   THE MANUFACTURERS' CALIBRATION STUDY

A.M.H.P. VAN DEN BESSELAAR and E.A. VAN DER VELDE

1. INTRODUCTION

Three certified Reference Materials (RMs) for thromboplastin are available from the Community Bureau of Reference (BCR) of the European Commission. These were prepared from different tissues, i.e. human brain (BCT/099), bovine brain (OBT/79) and rabbit brain (RBT/79). The RMs were calibrated against the primary WHO International Reference Preparation (coded 67/40) in an international collaborative study, in which seven European and three North-American laboratories participated (1,2,3).

In the present study these RMs were used by 12 manufacturers of commercially available thromboplastins for calibration of their products. Each manufacturer calibrated a representative batch of its production series (so-called house standard) against the RM that is most similar to the batch. Two manufacturers used two RMs and a third employed all three RMs. Two other manufacturers, each producing two different brands of thromboplastin, calibrated two corresponding house standards.

All manufacturers used a calibration protocol designed by a group of experts working with BCR (1,2,3). This protocol was recently adopted by WHO (6).

The group of experts working with BCR developed a new calibration model to relate prothrombin times (PTs) obtained with different thromboplastins. In essence, this model assumes a straight-line relationship, when the logarithms of PTs of normals and anticoagulated patients are plotted for one thromboplastin against the other. This model appeared to fulfill the requirements of accuracy in the calibration of the three RMs against the WHO International Reference Preparation 67/40.

The present report is an analysis of the calibration data obtained by the commercial manufacturers. The aim of this study is to test the new calibration model using the manufacturers' data. Furthermore, the precision of the calibration will be assessed.

2. DEFINITIONS

- Prothrombin Time Ratio: the prothrombin time of a patient under oral anticoagulant therapy divided by the mean prothrombin time of normal individuals using the same thromboplastin and same technique/technician.
- International Sensitivity Index (ISI): the slope of the orthogonal regression line when the logarithms of prothrombin times obtained with the primary International Reference Preparation (NIBSC code nr. 67/40) are plotted (y-axis) against the logarithms of prothrombin times obtained with a second thromboplastin on the same set of normals' and anticoagulated patients' plasmas.
- International Normalized Ratio (INR): a patient's prothrombin time ratio that is obtained using the primary International Reference Preparation (NIBSC code nr. 67/40), or the ratio that is calculated from measurements with a thromboplastin calibrated (directly or indirectly) against preparation 67/40. Such calculation may be conveniently done using the equation: $INR=R^{ISI}$, in which R is the ratio for the thromboplastin with known ISI.

3. RESULTS

3.1. Normal plasmas

Each manufacturer was requested to measure prothrombin times of 20 different fresh normal plasmas (besides 60 different fresh patient plasmas). Table 1 summarizes the data of the normals. The standard deviation comprises both biological and analytical variation. Each RM was used by several manufacturers. There are significant (one-way analysis of variance, $p<0.01$) differences between the laboratories that used the same RM. Furthermore, the

Table 1: Prothrombin times of normal individuals

RM = Reference Material

HS = House Standard

SD = Standard Deviation

Laboratory	Number of normals	RM used	Prothrombin time with RM		HS	Prothrombin time with HS	
			Mean (sec)	SD (sec)		Mean (sec)	SD (sec)
1	20	RBT/79	16.0	0.5	1	11.7	0.3
2	20	RBT/79	17.0	1.9	2	10.9	0.6
3	20	RBT/79	17.0	1.4	3	12.3	0.7
4	20	RBT/79	16.4	0.9	4	11.9	0.5
5	20	RBT/79	15.5	0.8	5	12.4	0.4
6	20	BCT/099	14.6	0.6	6	12.2	0.5
7	20	BCT/099	13.6	0.8	7	11.3	0.8
7	20	RBT/79	16.2	0.8			
8	20	BCT/099	12.9	0.3	8	14.1	0.2
8	20	OBT/79	35.5	0.7			
8	20	RBT/79	14.2	0.4			
9	20	OBT/79	38.4	2.3	9	39.8	2.1
10	20	RBT/79	16.5	1.0	10A	11.7	0.6
10	20				10B	13.9	0.9
11	19	OBT/79	39.0	4.3	11A	28.4	3.1
11	20	RBT/79	16.2	0.9	11B	34.7	1.8
12	18	RBT/79	16.3	1.4	12	12.4	0.9
12	15	BCT/099	14.7	1.1			

within-laboratory variation between the normals ranges from 2.7% (coefficient of variation) to 11.4%. It is interesting to note that laboratory 8, which used all three RMs, showed the lowest between-normal variation for all RMs, not only when compared with the other laboratories in this study, but also in comparison with the 7 European laboratories participating in the calibration of the three RMs versus 67/40 (1,2,3).

3.2. Patient plasmas

According to the calibration protocol, laboratories with access to a large number of patients were requested to select patients with prothrombin times within a range corresponding to 1.5-5 prolongation ratio in terms of the primary WHO Reference

Preparation 67/40. This range corresponds to:

    1.47 - 4.64 ratio (in terms of BCT/099)
    1.49 - 4.91 ratio (in terms of OBT/79)
    1.33 - 3.12 ratio (in terms of RBT/79)

Using the mean normal prothrombin time obtained by each laboratory, the number of patients lying outside the above-mentioned range was assessed (Table 2). Some laboratories differed a great deal when the anticoagulation levels of the patients were compared: 35% of the patients in laboratory 1 had INR values higher than 5.0; on the other hand, 27% of the patients in laboratory 9 had INR values lower than 1.5. Apparently, these laboratories had difficulties in obtaining patient samples with the required intensity of anticoagulation.

Table 2 Number of patients lying outside range of prothrombin time ratios corresponding to 1.5-5 International Normalized Ratio

Laboratory	RM used	total number of patients	number of patients with	
			INR < 1.5	INR > 5
1	RBT/79	60	–	21
2	RBT/79	60	3	2
3	RBT/79	60	1	2
4	RBT/79	60	1	9
5	RBT/79	60	1	–
6	BCT/099	53	5	1
7	BCT/099	60	4	–
7	RBT/79	60	6	1
8	BCT/099	60	3	1
8	OBT/79	60	2	1
8	RBT/79	60	2	1
9	OBT/79	55	15	1
10	RBT/79	60	–	20
11	OBT/79	59	1	12
11	RBT/79	60	1	20
12	RBT/79	69	1	18

3.3. Orthogonal regression lines of House Standards versus RMs

The new calibration model assumes a single straight-line relationship between the logarithms of prothrombin times of both normals and anticoagulated patients, when the results of one

Table 3 Test of the hypothesis of equal slopes and intercepts of the orthogonal regression lines through patients and normals separately. Tabulated are the p-values. Test for equal intercepts is only meaningful if slopes can be considered to be equal; for the four cases with p-value for slopes $\leq$ 0.05 the p-values for intercepts are given in brackets

| House standard | RM used for calibration | | | | | |
| | BCT/099 | | OBT/79 | | RBT/79 | |
	slope	intercept	slope	intercept	slope	intercept
1					0.557	0.132
2					0.003	(0.964)
3					0.812	0.194
4					1.000	0.000
5					0.912	0.587
6	0.929	0.099				
7	0.010	(0.325)			0.008	(0.462)
7*	0.589	0.717			0.701	0.150
8	0.004	(0.099)	0.573	0.073	0.111	0.002
9			0.127	0.273		
10A					0.353	0.015
10B					0.538	0.001
11A			0.920	0.073		
11A**			0.832	0.007		
11B					0.313	0.773
12	0.263	0.668			0.463	0.119

*After removal of one outlying normal
**After removal of one outlying patient

thromboplastin are plotted against the other. Figures 1 to 18 show the plots of logarithms of normal and patient PTs. It was tested whether the orthogonal regression lines through the normals and the patients coincide (4). In this analysis, it was tested first whether the lines have equal slopes. Next, it was tested whether the lines have equal intercepts, assuming that they have equal slopes. Table 3 gives the results of this analysis. In four cases the hypothesis of equal slopes was rejected. For laboratory 7, which used both RBT/79 and BCT/099, this rejection was due to one outlying normal value (see figures 7 and 8). After removal of this outlyer, the hypothesis of equal slopes was not rejected anymore.

Tables 4, 5 and 6 give the regression lines for the patient data only and for the combined data of patients and normals. In general, both lines are close to each other. The greatest differ-

Table 4 Orthogonal regression equations y = a + bx for house standard (x-axis) versus RBT/79 (y-axis). Data are in log
(time/s). s(a), s(b) and s are the standard deviations of a
and b, and the standard deviation about the regression line,
respectively.

House Standard	Patients				Patients plus normals				
	a	s(a)	b	s(b)	a	s(a)	b	s(b)	s
1	-.630	.104	1.691	.078	-.502	.033	1.596	.026	.016
2	-.088	.075	1.275	.060	-.131	.045	1.308	.037	.024
3	-.484	.096	1.555	.074	-.387	.043	1.481	.035	.018
4	-.451	.060	1.618	.047	-.769	.047	1.863	.038	.017
5	-.525	.107	1.578	.084	-.575	.040	1.617	.033	.013
7*	-.721	.168	1.817	.141	-.551	.075	1.677	.065	.022
8	-.518	.067	1.424	.048	-.358	.026	1.310	.020	.012
10A	-.797	.154	1.814	.113	-.498	.046	1.597	.035	.023
10B	-.244	.115	1.189	.071	.060	.032	1.003	.021	.030
11B	-.216	.098	.935	.050	-.243	.049	.948	.026	.038
12	-.276	.040	1.378	.029	-.322	.025	1.410	.019	.015

*after removal of one outlying normal

Table 5 Orthogonal regression equations y = a + bx for house standard (x-axis) versus BCT/099 (y-axis). Data are in log
(time/s). s(a), s(b) and s are the standard deviations, of a
and b, and the standard deviation about the regression line,
respectively

House Standard	Patients				Patients plus normals				
	a	s(a)	b	s(b)	a	s(a)	b	s(b)	s
6	.036	.056	1.061	.041	-.030	.032	1.107	.024	.018
7*	-1.053	.194	2.096	.162	-1.101	.091	2.136	.078	.022
8	-.851	.044	1.697	.031	-.795	.019	1.657	.014	.008
12	-.951	.147	1.952	.108	-.987	.085	1.978	.065	.035

*after removal of one outlying normal

ence in slope b is observed for house standard 10B, amounting to
about 18%. This is consistent with the observation that the lines
through patients and normals were different for this house standard (Table 3).

FIGURE 1-18. Prothrombin times (sec) obtained with the RM (y-axis) as a function of the prothrombin times (sec) obtained with each house standard (x-axis). Note the double-logarithmic scale. Data of normal plasmas are represented by circles and those of anticoagulated patients by triangles. Orthogonal regression lines are shown for patient data only and for the combined data of patients and normals. All data including outlyers are represented. The horizontal lines refer to anticoagulation intensities corresponding to 1.5 INR and 5.0 INR.

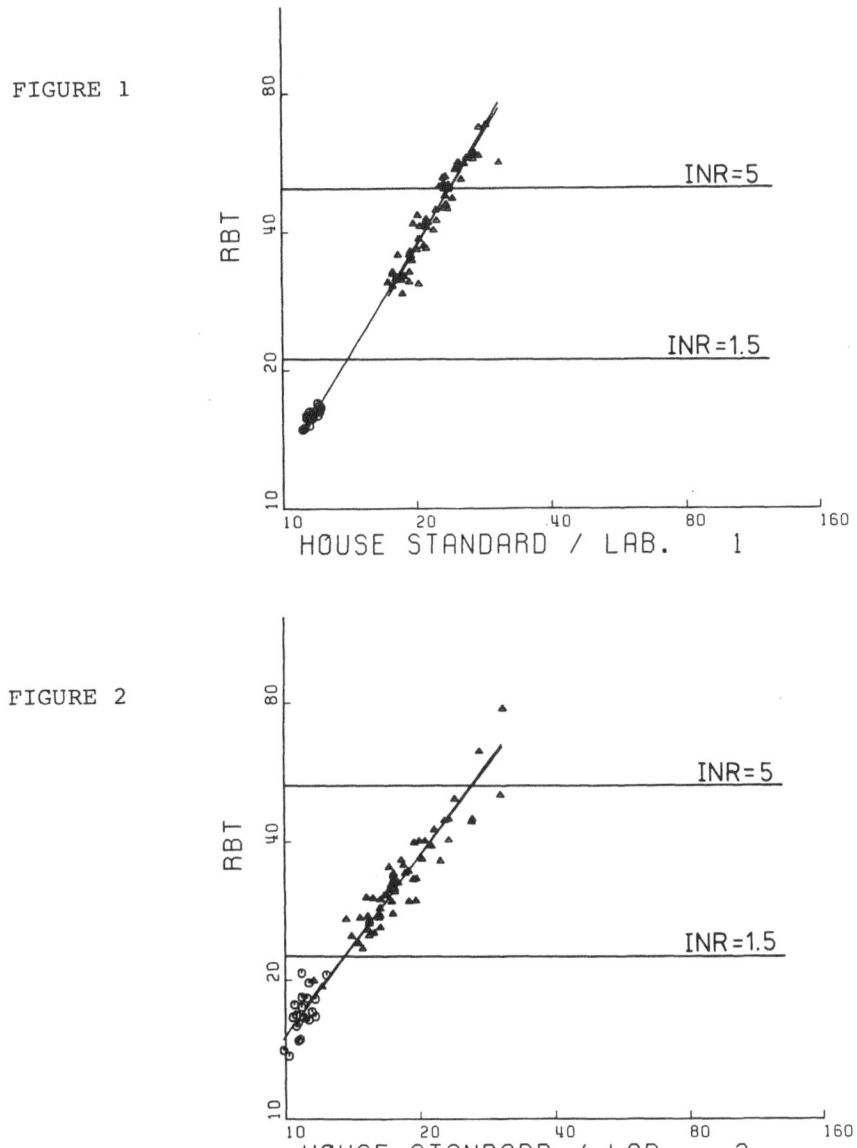

FIGURE 3

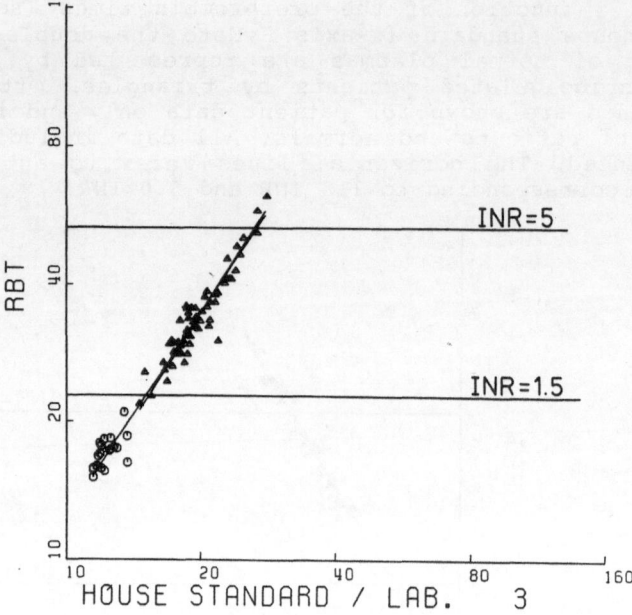

FIGURE 4

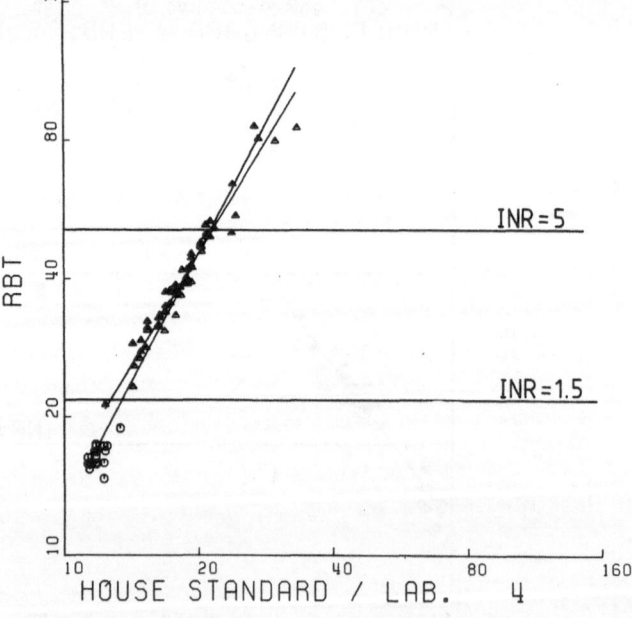

FIGURE 5

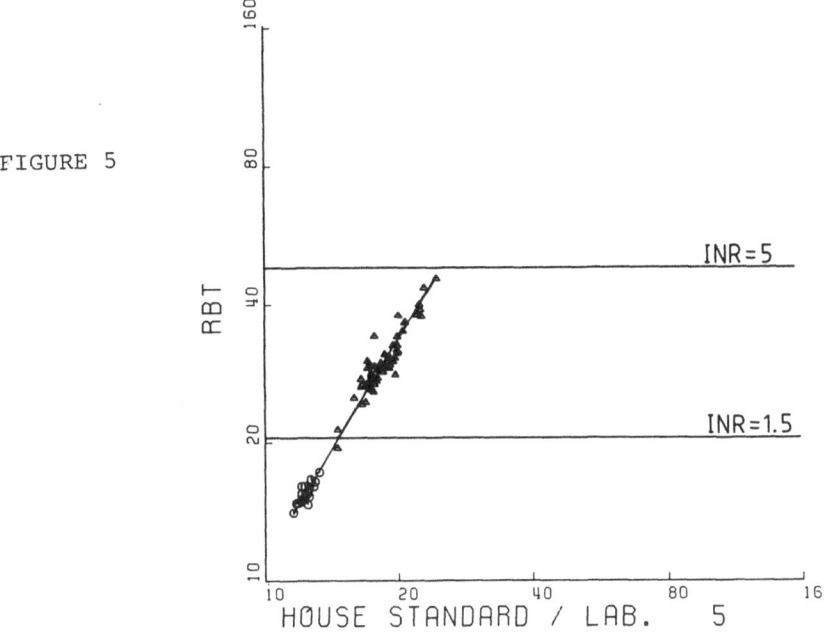

HOUSE STANDARD / LAB.   5

FIGURE 6

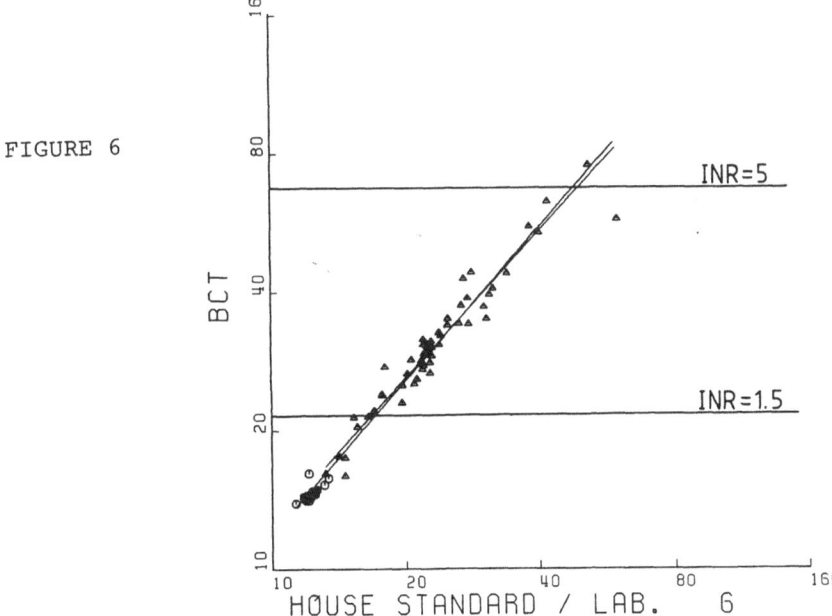

HOUSE STANDARD / LAB.   6

FIGURE 7

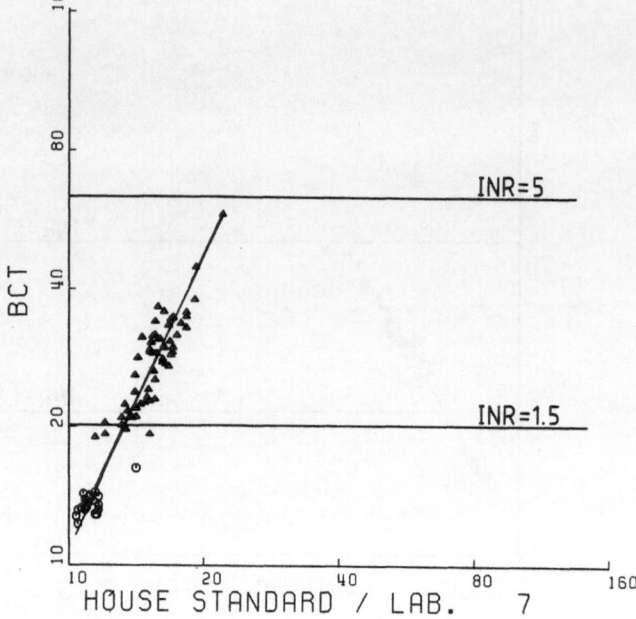

FIGURE 8

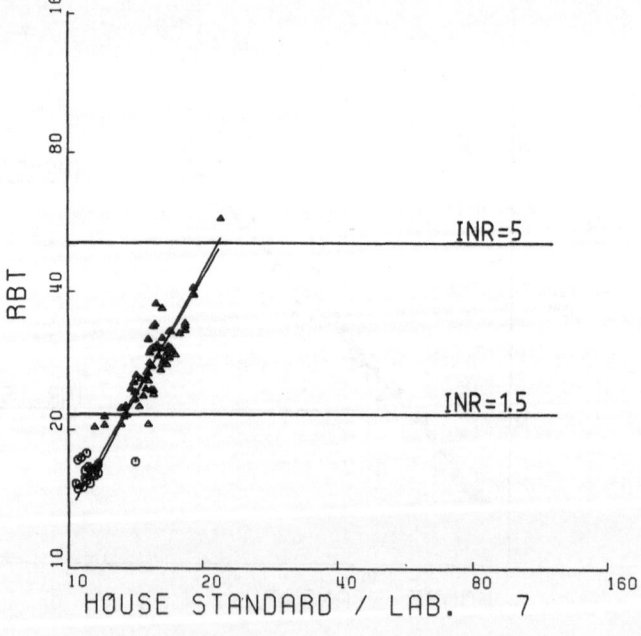

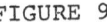

FIGURE 9

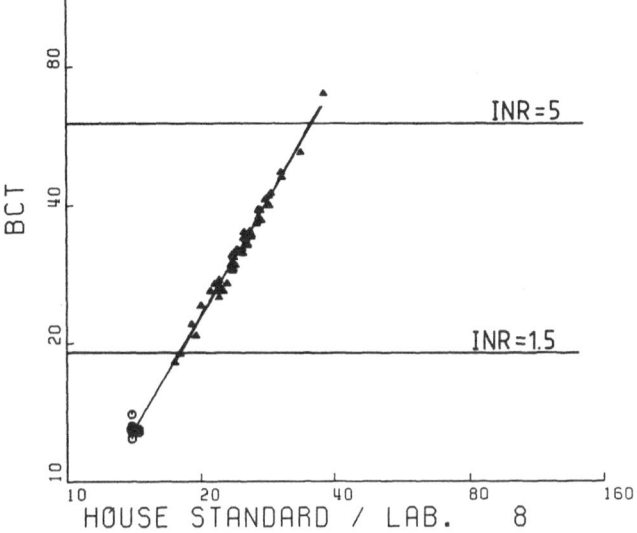

IGURE 10

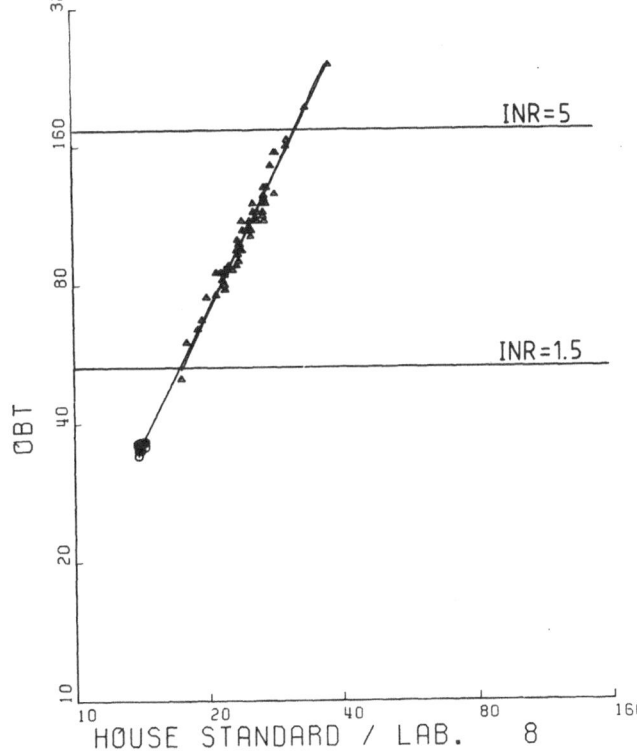

138

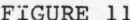

FIGURE 11

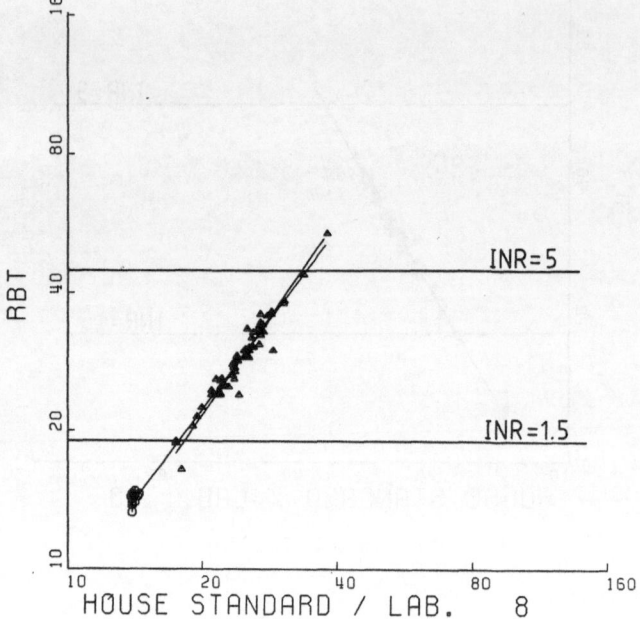

FIGURE 12

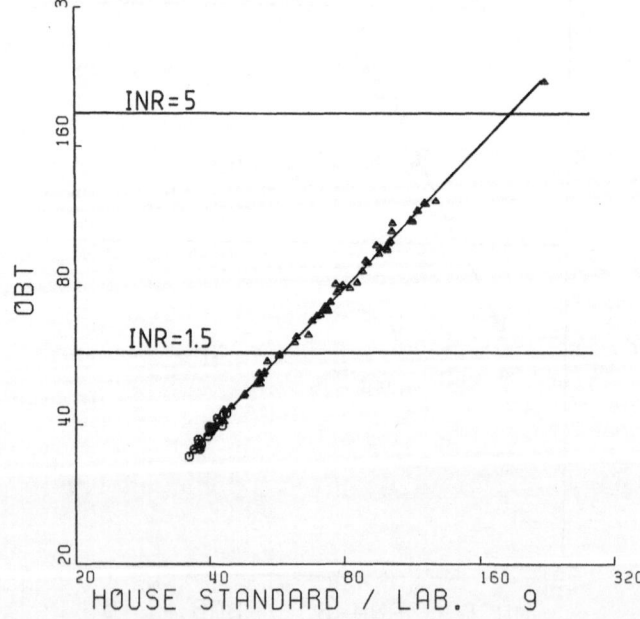

FIGURE 13

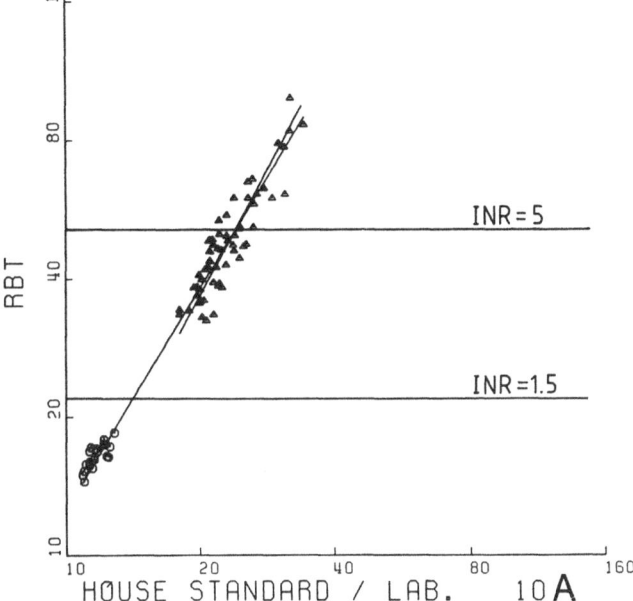

FIGURE 14

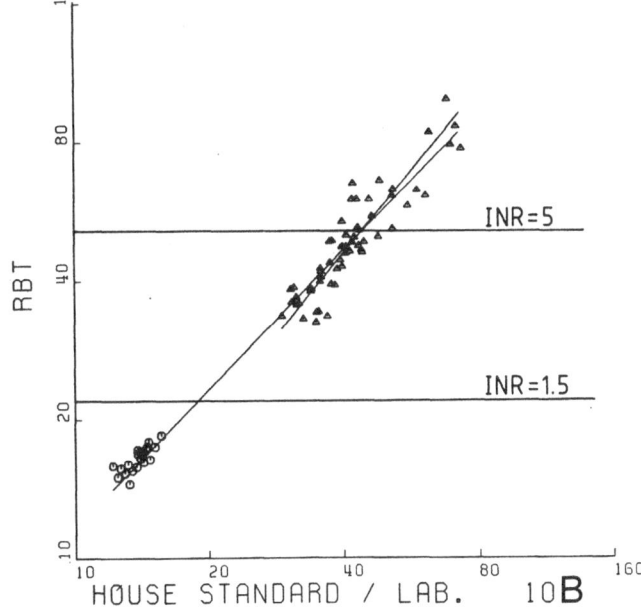

140

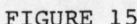

FIGURE 15

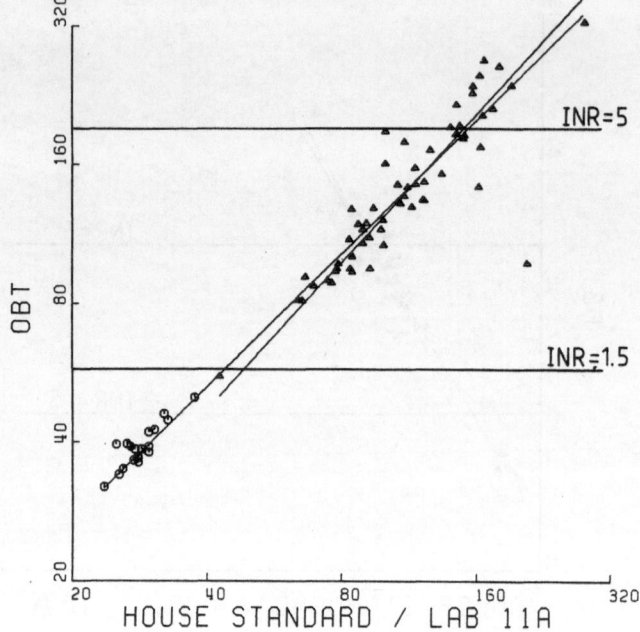

FIGURE 16

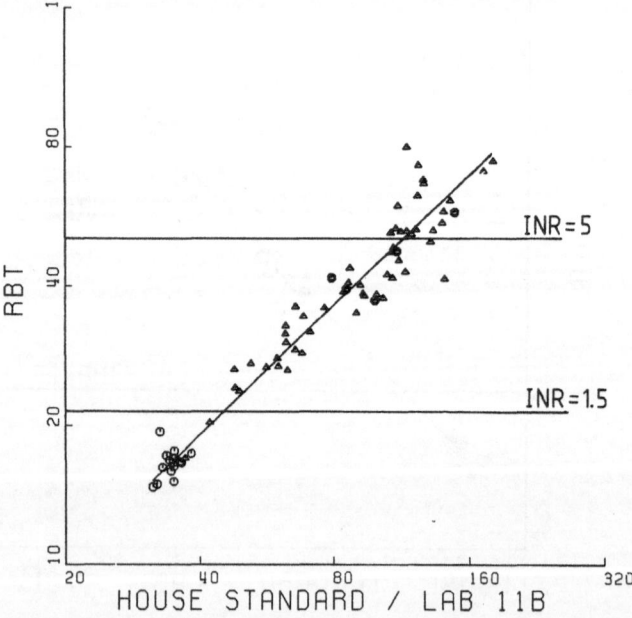

FIGURE 17

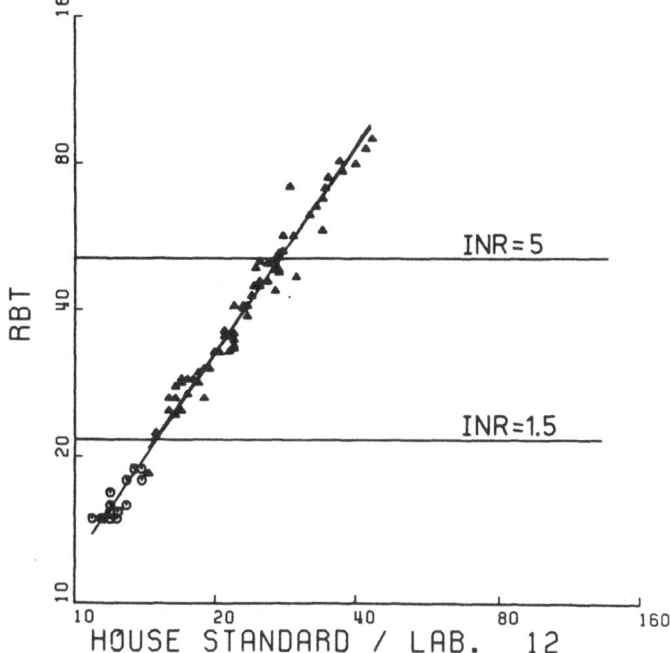

FIGURE 18

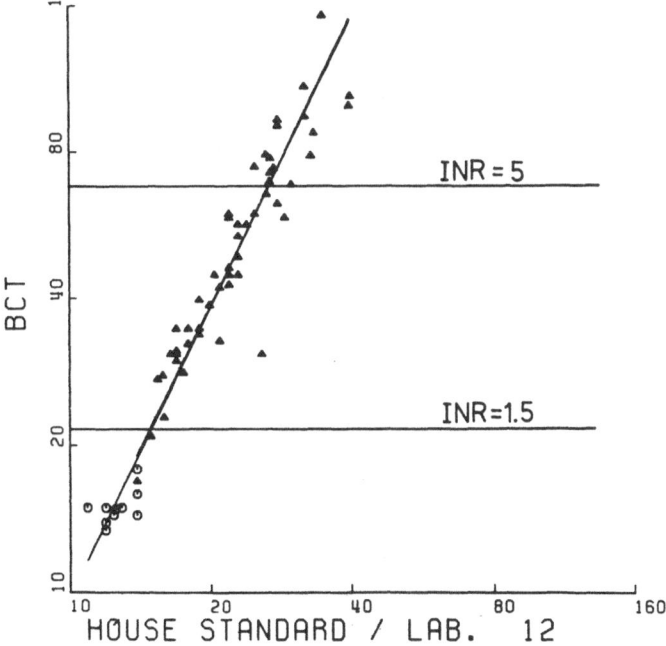

Table 6 Orthogonal regression equations y = a + bx for house standard (x-axis) versus OBT/79 (y-axis). Data are in
log(time/s). s(a), s(b) and s are the standard deviations of
a and b, and the standard deviation about the regression
line respectively.

House Standard	Patients				Patients plus normals				
	a	s(a)	b	s(b)	a	s(a)	b	s(b)	s
8	-.785	.070	2.014	.050	-.686	.027	1.943	.020	.010
9	-.036	.019	1.015	.010	-.053	.012	1.024	.007	.007
11A	-.032	.161	1.064	.078	.183	.054	.961	.028	.050
11A*	-.064	.108	1.084	.053	.161	.039	.975	.020	.036

*After removal of one outlying patient

4. DISCUSSION

An important aim of thromboplastin calibration is to establish
equivalent therapeutic ranges of oral anticoagulation. The precision and accuracy of such ranges are directly dependent on those
of the calibration. We will now consider the variability of the
individual data (the scatter of the points in the calibration
plot) and the validity of the mathematical model used to describe
the calibration relationship.

The variation of the individual data, which comprises both
biological and experimental variation, is reflected in the standard deviation of slope b and intercept a, and more importantly,
in the standard deviation about the orthogonal regression line.
The standard deviations of a and b not only depend on biological
and experimental variation, but also on the distribution of the
samples. The most direct measure of biological and experimental
variation is the standard deviation (s) about the regression
line. The value for s is very low for house standard 9, probably
because this house standard is very similar to the RM used for
calibration (Table 6). On the other hand, the value for s is
relatively large for house standards 11A and 11B (Tables 4 and
6), which might be related to the dissimilarity of the RMs used.

The mathematical model used in this study assumes a straight-
line relationship between the logarithms of the prothrombin times

of normals and patients. In the previous section we have seen
that in some cases a significant deviation from this model occurs. From these observations one may conclude that the relationship is curved instead of rectilinear. This implies that if the
rectilinear model is applied to these data, the resulting regression line parameters are dependent on the level of anticoagulation. This aspect should be investigated more thoroughly because
we have seen that some laboratories have used patients with very
different levels of anticoagulation (see Table 2).

Table 7 Effect of anticoagulation intensity on orthogonal regression
equation y = a + bx for house standard 4 (x-axis) versus
RBT/79 (y-axis).
Data are in log(time/s).

number of normals	number of patients	mean patient ratio (RBT/79)	slope b	intercept a
–	60	2.46	1.62	-.451
20	60	2.46	1.86	-.769
20	33*	2.00	2.05	-.977
20	50**	2.28	1.98	-.899

*patients with INR ≤ 3.5 only
**patients with INR ≤ 5.0 only

Most patient plasmas used by laboratory 7 (58 out of 60) had
PT ratios with RBT/79 smaller than 2.4 (INR≈3.5). In contrast,
laboratory 4 had only 33 patients with RBT ratios smaller than
2.4. The calibration model used in this study was not completely
appropriate to describe the relationship between the house standard of laboratory 4 and RBT/79 (Table 3). We have calculated the
regression line for laboratory 4 using the normals and the patients with RBT ratios smaller than 2.4, i.e., patients with an
anticoagulation level similar to that of virtually all patients
used by laboratory 7 (Table 7). In addition, a regression line
was calculated using the normals and the patients with INR≤5. By
using only the relatively weakly anticoagulated patients
(INR≤3.5) the slope of the orthogonal regression line is increased from 1.86 to 2.05. Table 8 gives a comparison of the

equivalent ratios calculated with four different regression lines, i.e., the line for all patients without the normals, the line for all patients plus normals, the line for the normals plus the low-intensity patients (INR≤3.5), and the line for the normals plus patients with INR≤5. The calculations were performed according to the pathway shown on the right side of Figure 19.

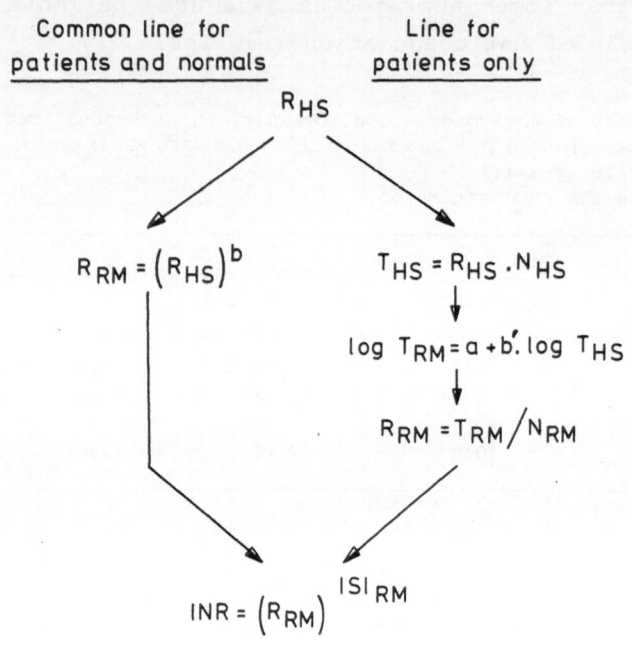

FIGURE 19. Two alternative pathways for transformation of ratios with a house standard (R_{HS}) into International Normalized Ratios (INR). b is the slope of the orthogonal regression line for the combined patients' and normals' data. b' is the slope of the line for the patients only. T and N are the prothrombin times of patients and normals, respectively.

It is clear that the level of anticoagulation of patients used for calibration has an important effect on the equivalent ratios of house standard and International Reference Preparation. The difference between the calculated INR values may amount to about 15% (Table 8). The difference is minimal in the middle of the therapeutic range (INR≈3).

Table 8 Equivalent prothrombin time ratios calculated with different orthogonal regression lines (see Table 7). R_{HS} is the ratio for House Standard 4.
Calculation of INRs is done according to the pathway on the right in Figure 19.

Regression line used	INR value (calculated)			
	$R_{HS}=1.1$	$R_{HS}=1.3$	$R_{HS}=1.5$	$R_{HS}=1.8$
60 patients	1.58	2.32	3.22	4.88
60 patients + 20 normals	1.37	2.13	3.10	5.01
33 patients* + 20 normals	1.35	2.19	3.30	5.60
50 patients** + 20 normals	1.37	2.19	3.27	5.45

*patients with INR ≤ 3.5 only
**patients with INR ≤ 5.0 only

The selection of patient samples for determination of the calibration line deserves a further comment. If patient samples are selected as to anticoagulation intensity using the prothrombin times for the RM only, a systematic underestimation of the slope of the orthogonal regression line is likely to result, because of the random variation of individual assessments about the regression line. The prothrombin times assessed with the thromboplastin to be calibrated should also be taken into account. Therefore, if patient samples are to be selected within the 1.5-5 INR range, the cut-off lines should be drawn perpendicularly to the orthogonal regression line for all data points, as illustrated in Figure 20.

The RMs were calibrated against the WHO International Reference Preparation 67/40 in an international collaborative study. Combination of the calibration parameters obtained in that study with the present house standard calibration allows us to compare equivalent ratios (Table 9). Calibration of a given house standard against different RMs should result in identical equivalent ratios. This is indeed observed for the laboratories that used more than one RM. For laboratory 7 and 12 there is excellent agreement between the ratios calculated via BCT/099 and RBT/79. For laboratory 8, the equivalent ratios corresponding to 5 INR vary a little more but are still reasonably close to each other.

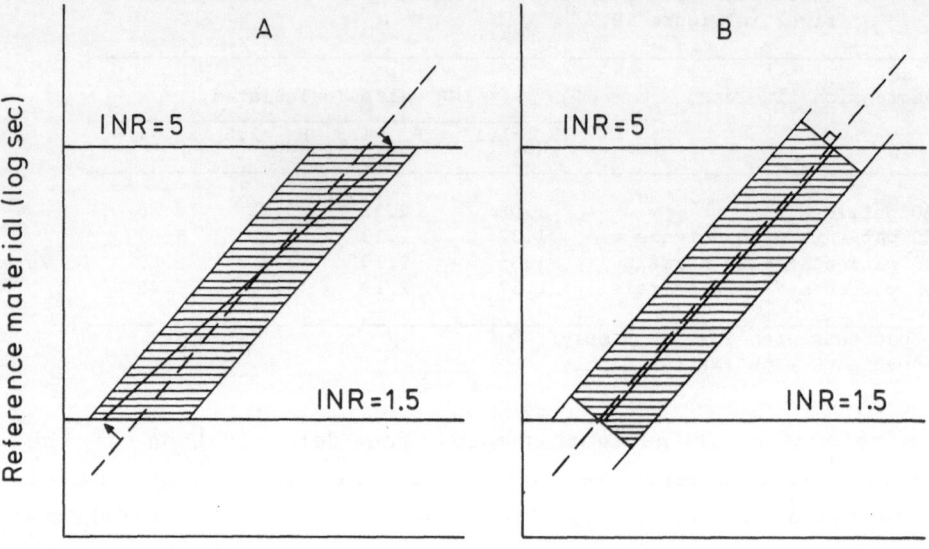

FIGURE 20. Selection of patient samples within 1.5–5.0 INR range. The shaded areas represent the scatter of the individual patient data points. The interrupted line is the orthogonal regression line for all patient data.
Left figure (A): if the cut-off lines are drawn parallel to the horizontal axis, the orthogonal regression line for the selected samples will be slightly biased.
Right figure (B): if the cut-off lines are drawn perpendicular to the regression line for all patient data, no bias will result.

Table 9 shows a comparison of two ways in which equivalent ratios can be calculated. The first method is a consequence of the calibration model in which it is assumed that both normals and patients comply with a single rectilinear relationship in the logarithms of the prothrombin times. This assumption leads to the simple equation: $\log(INR) = ISI \cdot \log(R)$. The second method assumes that the logarithms of only patients' prothrombin times comply with a rectilinear relationship. Both calculation methods are shown in Figure 19. For most house standards, there is excellent

agreement between both methods (Table 9). Relatively large discrepancies are observed for house standards 4, 10A, 10B and 11A
at the lower limit of the equivalent range (INR=1.5) due to inadequacy of the BCR/WHO model. It may well be that this discrepancy is of minor clinical importance and that the BCR/WHO
model is suitable in clinical practice also for these house standards. Furthermore, the discrepancies are much smaller at the
other side of the range (INR=5).

Table 9 International Sensitivity Index (ISI) and equivalent ratios
for house standards

House Standard	RM used for calibration	ISI (1)	Ratios corresponding to 1.5-5.0 INR	
			according to INR = R^{ISI}	according to regression line for patients only (2)
1	RBT/79	2.26	1.20-2.04	1.24-2.04
2	RBT/79	1.85	1.25-2.39	1.24-2.41
3	RBT/79	2.09	1.21-2.16	1.24-2.15
4	RBT/79	2.63	1.17-1.84	1.07-1.82
5	RBT/79	2.28	1.19-2.02	1.19-2.03
6*	BCT/099	1.20	1.40-3.83	1.39-3.84
7**	BCT/099	2.24	1.20-2.05	1.18-2.05
7**	RBT/79	2.37	1.19-1.97	1.20-1.92
8	BCT/099	1.74	1.26-2.53	1.28-2.51
8	OBT/79	1.96	1.23-2.27	1.25-2.26
8	RBT/79	1.85	1.24-2.39	1.29-2.36
9	OBT/79	1.03	1.48-4.74	1.47-4.75
10A	RBT/79	2.26	1.20-2.04	1.29-2.06
10B	RBT/79	1.42	1.33-3.11	1.55-3.17
11A*	OBT/79	0.99	1.51-5.08	1.71-5.15
11B	RBT/79	1.34	1.35-3.32	1.31-3.27
12	RBT/79	1.99	1.23-2.25	1.19-2.21
12	BCT/099	2.07	1.22-2.18	1.20-2.15

(1). ISI was calculated according to the equation: $ISI=(b.ISI_{RM})$
in which ISI_{RM} is given by the BCR certificate (3) and b is
the slope of the orthogonal regression line calculated for patients plus normals (given in Tables 4, 5, or 6)
(2). see pathway on the right in Figure 19

* one outlying patient has been removed
** one outlying normal has been removed

In this contribution the hypothesis was tested that the lines
for the normals and for the patients coincide. An alternative

approach was employed by Tomenson (5), who argued that it is sufficient to demonstrate that the mean logarithms of the pro-thrombin times of normals lie on the orthogonal regression line for the patients' plasmas. The latter approach is more straight-forward with respect to the applicability of the equation INR = antilog(ISI·logR). This is shown in the case of house standard 2, where the slopes of normals' and patients' lines are significantly different (Table 3), but both calculation pathways in Figure 19 yield virtually the same INRs (Table 9). This is because in this case the mean of normals lies on the patients' line (Figure 2). However, in Tomenson's test (5) a difference in slope between patients' and normals' line may remain undetected. When the slopes are different, the standard deviation about the regression line of the combined patients' and normals' data could be larger than the standard deviation about the separate lines.

5. CONCLUSIONS

This study has shown that manufacturers of commercial thrombo-plastins can perform calibration of their house standards accor-ding to the BCR/WHO protocol. It became apparent that there are important differences between the anticoagulant intensities aimed at in the clinics providing the samples for calibration. Some clinics have a substantial proportion of their patients beyond the 1.5-5 INR range, the latter range being recommended for cali-bration. For most house standards, the calibration model advoca-ted by BCR/WHO is valid. For a few house standards, a statisti-cally significant deviation from this model was found, which may not be clinically important in all cases.

REFERENCES

1. Hermans J, Van den Besselaar AMHP, Loeliger EA, Van der Velde EA. A collaborative calibration study of reference materials for thromboplastins. Thromb Haemostas 1983; 50:712-717.
2. Hermans J. The European Community Bureau of Reference Cali-bration Study. This volume, chapter 4.
3. Loeliger EA, Van den Besselaar AMHP, Hermans J, Van der Velde EA. Certification of three reference materials for thrombo-plastins. BCR information. Commission of the European Commu-nities, Brussels 1981.

4. Van der Velde EA, Orthogonal regression equation. This volume, chapter 3.
5. Tomenson JA. A statistician's independent evaluation. This volume, chapter 5.
6. WHO Expert Committee on Biological Standardization. 33rd Report. WHO Technical Report Series, 687: pp. 81-105. WHO, Geneva 1983.

Chapter 8:   INR RANGES AND TARGETS FOR ORAL ANTICOAGULATION TO
BE EFFECTIVE AND SAFE

E.A. LOELIGER

After the contribution by Van den Besselaar and Van der Velde
(Chapter 7), two clinical questions urge themselves upon the
reader. First, why these wide differences in intensity of anticoagulation of the patients whose plasmas were used for thromboplastin calibration? And second: what is the relationship between
intensity of anticoagulation and its clinical effectiveness and
risks?

Figure 1 illustrates recommendations of therapeutic ranges,
those represented in <u>black</u> bars originating from data presented
by the manufacturers in the package inserts accompanying the
thromboplastin preparations, and those represented in <u>hatched</u>
bars being recommended since 1977 by Prof. Duckert of Basel
University (1,2). On the horizontal axis, the International
Normalized Ratios (INRs) are given, that are ratios with the
International Reference Preparation calculated from the prothrombin time ratio using a thromboplastin with a known International
Sensitivity Index (ISI). (The INRs were calculated from ratios or
percentages using, where needed, the (mostly linear) relationship
of the inverse of the percentages with the prothrombin times, in
French called the Thivolle relationship. The formula for translation is: $INR = R^{ISI}$, the ISI being taken from the manufacturers' house standard calibration study (10)).

The scale limits presented in Figure 1 also deserve explanation. The broken line at the left-hand side marks the lower
minimum level of anticoagulation, that is an INR of 1.5, to be
observed for instance in patients on coumarin prophylaxis under-
going neurosurgical procedures. The broken line at the right-hand
side marks the upper limit of the therapeutic range, that is an

152

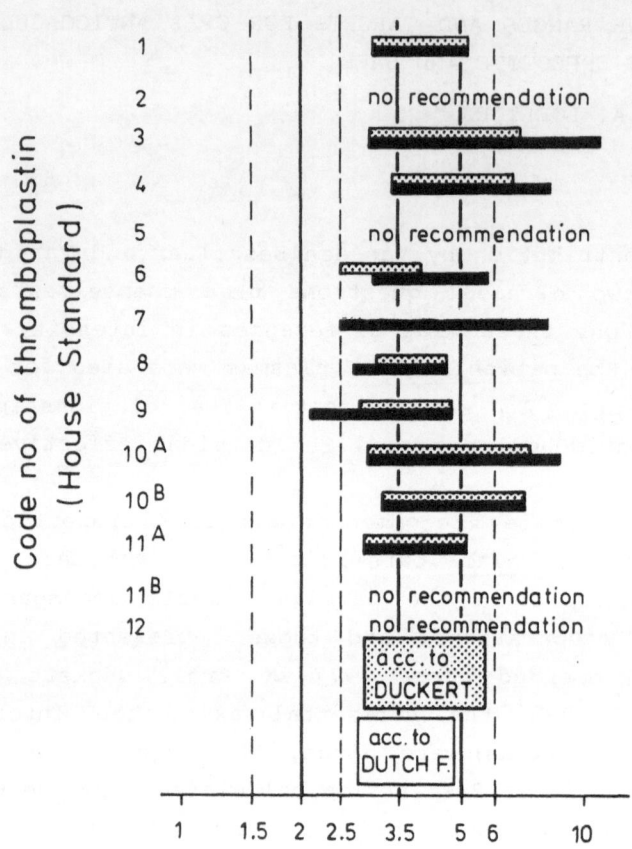

FIGURE 1: Recommended therapeutic ranges for various thromboplastins translated into INRs. The code numbers refer to the
thromboplastins used in the Manufacturers' Calibration Study
(10). Black bars refer to recommendations made by the manufacturers and hatched bars to those made by Duckert (1). The
recommended values were translated into INR using the equation
INR = antilog(ISI·log R), where R is the prothrombin time ratio
and ISI the slope of the calibration line, the latter obtained
from the Manufacturers' Calibration Study (10). It should be
noted that any errors in the ISI values are transmitted also to
ranges recommended by Duckert (1). At the bottom of the figure,
the average recommendation by Duckert (1) and the recommendation
by the Federation of Dutch Thrombosis Centres are given.

INR of 6, being, in our experience, the upper maximum tolerable limit for patients with artificial heart valves in whom the target intensity of the Leiden Centre approximates an INR of 4.5 (3). The usual range adopted by the Dutch Federation of Thrombosis Services, marked at the bottom of the figure, is for active venous thrombosis and for arterial indications 2.8-4.8 INR, with a target of 3.5 INR (4), the latter marked by a bold vertical line. For cases with contra-indications, the lower limit is 2.2 INR, and the target 2.9 INR.

In Prof. Duckert's publications (1,2), the 15-25 per cent range for home-made human brain thromboplastin was given as the range in relation to which those of all other thromboplastins were calculated. On closer scrutiny, the Thrombotest range equivalent to 15-25 per cent home-made human brain thromboplastin was not exactly 5-10% but 4.6-9.5%, as Prof. Duckert told me by letter in June 1983. Hence, Prof. Duckert's recommendations, as indicated at the bottom of Figure 1, reflect a slightly more intensive anticoagulation than those adopted by the Dutch Federation of Thrombosis Services, holding for patients suffering from venous or arterial thrombosis without contra-indications and corresponding to 2.8-4.8 INR.

Looking at Figure 1 and considering unprejudiced the limits presented, the most eye-catching feature is perhaps that none of the manufacturers refers to clinical situations where patients have to, or may be kept at levels between 1.5 and 2.5 INR with a target INR of 2, values recently recommended by the Hamilton group for venous prophylaxis in discharged patients after hospitalization for acute venous thrombosis (5) and by the Mayo Clinics for per-operative anticoagulation (6). The second striking feature is that the manufacturers of thromboplastins 3, 4, 7, 10A, and 10B surpass the Dutch safety limit of 6 INR, referred to a moment ago. These manufacturers recommend to keep patients at levels up to or even more than 10 INR.

With respect to the second question, namely that concerning the relationship between the intensity of anticoagulation and the bleeding risk, I would like to remind you that Dutch recommendations are based on well-controlled retrospective data for many tens of thousands of patient treatment years annually, recommendations validated by the randomized double-blind prospective 60-Plus Reinfarction Study, performed under the auspices of the Federation in the late seventies (4). In the more than 500 elderly patients of this trial, hospitalization for major extracranial bleeding, in my view the strongest criterion of the risk of long-term oral anticoagulation, occurred once in 70 years at risk. The study was performed under the conditions of a target INR of 3.5 and with more than 70 per cent of the INRs lying between 2.8 and 4.8 (4). The second best parameter of the tendency to bleed under oral anticoagulation is, in my view, the incidence of macro-haematuria. Figure 2 demonstrates the incidence of macrohaematuria, presented logarithmically in per cent per year at risk on the y-axis, in relation to the intensity of anticoagulation in terms of INR linearly on the x-axis. The well-controlled data strongly suggest an exponential augmentation of the incidence, steeply increasing with increasing intensity of anticoagulation. The lowest incidence was observed by Forfar (7), who published his findings in patients kept at a low intensity, the target lying between 2-2.5 British Ratios which are virtually identical with INRs, a range which was customary in the sixties and early seventies in Britain and as has been shown by Taberner and Poller to be safe in the per-operative period in major gynaecological surgery (8). The highest incidence was scored by the Rotterdam Thrombosis Centre, where more than 7,500 patients are under supervision continuously, with the highest intensity of anticoagulation among Dutch thrombosis centres. It is important to notice that the incidence observed in the prospective 60-Plus Study represented by the black dot in about the middle of all symbols is neatly on line with the retrospective data - our overall conclusion is that under conditions of intensity and stability of anticoagulation as applied by the majority of Centres in The Netherlands, the incidence of macro-haematuria in the population of Dutch thrombosis services, of which 60 to 70 per cent of individuals suffer from atherothrombotic diseases, is roughly ten times the incidence in the non-anticoagulated population. Interestingly, the third not easily biassed parameter, i.e., the incidence of <u>intracranial haemorrhage</u>, is, as evidenced for elderly patients on long-term oral anticoagulation, according to Dutch standards, similarly increased to about ten times that of the control group (9,11).

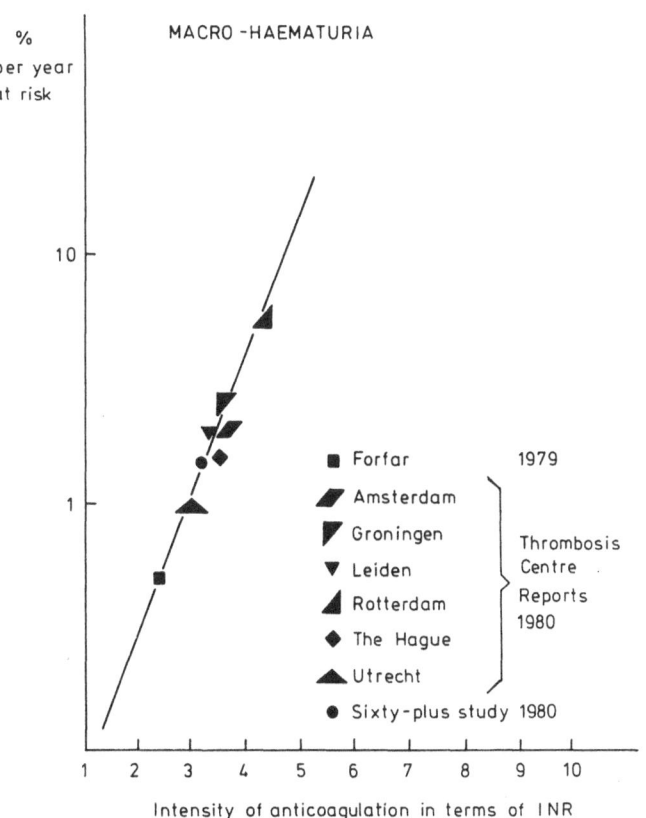

FIGURE 2: Relationship between anticoagulation intensity (expressed as International Normalized Ratio in a linear scale) and incidence of macro-haematuria as reported by the centres referred to in the figure. The percentage of patients per year with a bleeding episode is represented on a logarithmic scale (vertical axis). A straight line through the data points reflects the relationship reasonably well.

Looking at Figure 2 once again, it is tempting to extrapolate the bleeding incidence to patients kept at INRs between 5 and 10. Table 1 shows the result of extrapolation: at a target of 10 INR, the incidence of major haemorrhage would amount to 1/week!

Although this probably is an overestimation, it points to the
high risk of bleeding if patients are kept at levels of intensity
near the upper limit as recommended and obviously considered to
be clinically acceptable by the advisors of the manufacturers of
thromboplastins 3, 4, 7, 10A, and 10B.

Table 1

INR	Risk of major bleeding per year (elderly population)
2	1 : 250
3.5	1 : 50
4.7	1 : 10
6	1 : 2.5
7.5	1 : 0.5
10	1 : 0.02

In sum: the recommendations for the limits of therapeutic
anticoagulation made by about half of the manufacturers of the
thromboplastins under study - marking the 2.5-5 INR range - are
in good agreement with Prof. Duckert's recommendations based on
Dutch and Swiss experience. These recommendations hold for active
venous thrombosis and arterial indications, but obviously reflect
excessively strong anticoagulation for simple venous prophylaxis.
Experts recommending intensities of INRs > 6 insufficiently
recognize the bleeding risk accompanying such intensity. Manufacturers of thromboplastins are urged to reconsider, in the light
of the results and discussions of the present House Standard
Calibration Study (10), their recommendations with respect to
optimal therapeutic ranges and to make revisions where needed.

REFERENCES

1. Duckert F, Marbet GA. Die Kontrolle der oralen Antikoagula-
    tion. Der therapeutische Bereich. Schweiz Rundschau Med
    (Praxis) 1977; 66: 293-294.
2. Duckert F, Marbet GA. Le contrôle du traitement aux anticoa-
    gulants oraux. La zone thérapeutique. Méd et Hyg 1977; 35:
    911.

3. Loeliger EA. Oral anticoagulants and/or aspirin. In: Roskamm H (ed.), Prognosis of coronary heart disease - Progression of coronary arteriosclerosis, Springer Verlag, Heidelberg 1983: pp. 223-230.
4. Sixty Plus Reinfarction Study Research Group. A double-blind trial to assess long-term oral anticoagulant therapy in elderly patients after myocardial infarction. Lancet 1980; 2: 989-994.
5. Hull R, Hirsh J, Carter C et al. Different intensities of oral anticoagulant therapy in the treatment of proximal-vein thrombosis. N Engl J Med 1982; 307: 1676-1681.
6. Francis CW, Marder VJ, Evarts CMcC et al. Two-step warfarin therapy. J Amer Med Ass 1983; 249: 374-378.
7. Forfar JC. A 7-year analysis of haemorrhage in patients on long-term anticoagulant treatment. Br Heart J 1979; 42: 128-132.
8. Taberner DA, Poller L, Burslem RW, Jones JB. Oral anticoagulants controlled by the British comparative thromboplastin versus low-dose heparin in prophylaxis of deep vein thrombosis. Br Med J 1978; 1: 272-274.
9. Sixty-Plus Reinfarction Study Research Group. Risks of long-term oral anticoagulant therapy in elderly patients after myocardial infarction. Lancet 1982; 1: 64-68.
10. Van den Besselaar AMHP, Van der Velde EA. The manufacturers' calibration study. This volume, chapter 7.
11. Wintzen AR, De Jonge H, Loeliger EA, Bots GTAM. The risk of intracerebral haemorrhage during oral anticoagulant treatment: a population study. Ann Neurol, accepted for publication 1983.

DISCUSSION

Chairmen: R.M. BERTINA
         J.A. KOEPKE

SPAETHE: The results are very much influenced by the type of anticoagulation of the patient. When you have a highly anticoagulated patient, the result is differently influenced than with a low degree of anticoagulation. Is it correct that the calibration comparison between reagents is better, with a lower range of anticoagulation?

VAN DEN BESSELAAR: It is possible that in the high intensity anticoagulation range, the WHO model becomes invalid and you get a curvature of the double-logarithmic plot.

LOELIGER: The patients in our thrombosis service in whom the INR values are higher than 6, are in general destabilized, and such outliers will also bias the calibration line.

DENSON: I think we go back to the question of PIVKA. If you are dealing with dissimilar materials, PIVKA sensitive and PIVKA insensitive, then the calibration is quite definitely going to depend on the degree of anticoagulation. But when you are talking about manufacturers' batch production of like material, I don't think it matters. Another point is that I don't think we have completely exhausted the idea of using normal plasma and adsorbed normal plasma as standards for calibration, in other words to get out of coumarin plasma altogether. The ICTH/ICSH study showed that when you came to look at dissimilar thromboplastins, there was gross discrepancy. I am sure that for rabbit brain it is possible to do batch calibration with normal plasma and adsorbed plasma.

BERTINA: What must be done when the regression lines through the patients' data points and the normal points are not identical? What decisions have to be made by the manufacturer?

VAN DEN BESSELAAR: In the case where the patients' line deviates from the line through the combined data of patients and normals (as was observed for house standard 4 in the Manufacturers' Calibration Study), it is not appropriate to assign an ISI value to the thromboplastin in question, because this would introduce a bias. This bias is relatively large at low anticoagulation intensity and becomes increasingly less at higher intensities.

In that case the manufacturer should not provide an ISI, but only a table or a chart relating INRs to ratios with the house standard or the batch.

KIRKWOOD: There are two alternative answers to this question. The first is to accept that you use a system which does not exactly fit the data. Although there is evidence that it is not statistically correct, you nevertheless fit a line through the mean of the normals and the patients. You accept that you introduce thereby a small bias. It is a matter for clinicians to decide whether this bias is acceptable. If the procedure is acceptable, it has the advantage that even though there will be a few rare instances where manufacturers' preparations don't exactly fit the calibration model, you still keep exactly the same terminology and exactly the same principle. The alternative is as dr. Van den Besselaar indicated, to prepare a conversion chart which is not directly found in the WHO scheme, but may be regarded as a special case for the particular instance. The choice must be guided by the clinical implications of the alternatives. It is whether you use, for the sake of convenience, a system which is not exactly perfect and introduces a small bias, or whether you make an exception in this instance and prepare something special.

BERTINA: Do you think that this type of discrepancy is linked to special combinations of thromboplastins? Or is it something that may occur only in some of the batches of one type of thromboplastin?

VAN DEN BESSELAAR: At present we have too few data to confirm this. We should study a thromboplastin such as no. 4 in more detail and calibrate it against several types of thromboplastin to see whether this deviation of the patients' line from the normals is present in each case.

LOELIGER: With respect to house standard no. 4, we have seen that a 1.4 INR, which is outside the clinically relevant range, was deviating 13%, while at INR = 3 it was less than 5%, and at INR = 5 it was even less than 3%. From the clinical point of view, such differences are negligible. In my view, thromboplastin no 4 would work very well in our centre, if we would have a need for replacement of our actual thromboplastin.

VAN DER VELDE: Dr. Kirkwood mentioned two possibilities for handling situations where the thromboplastin does not fit into the system because of the patients' line not going through the normals. There is a third possibility, which is not to produce that thromboplastin any longer.

KOEPKE: There is an example of this in the United States. A number of years ago, when we first looked at prothrombin times in the CAP surveys, we found some thromboplastins which did not seem to be acting like they should. For one reason or another those dropped out of the market and some of them also changed significantly.

DENSON: These should be guidelines, and I hope ultimately, that we will have proficiency testing and quality control. Whatever the manufacturer puts to the slope of the line, and whatever the standard error is, the proof of the pudding will be in what is obtained at the bench for an INR. This will surely show in proficiency testing and quality control. If a product is no good or has the wrong slope, it will be discarded.

Table 1: INR equivalents of survey plasmas (Etalonorme, 1981)

| | adsorbed | | coumadinized | |
	E_3	F_3	E_4	F_4
bioMérieux (rabbit)	2.3 (270)*	3.3 (287)*	3.3 (270)*	2.3 (287)*
Stago (rabbit/simian)	2.3 (202)	3.3 (245)	3.5 (202)	2.5 (245)
Techn. Biol. (rabbit?)	2.3 (78)	3.3 (59)	3.5 (78)	2.5 (59)
Thrombotest (bovine)	1.9 (473)	2.5 (169)	3.2 (434)	2.5 (168)

ISI (RELAC) bioM 2.2; St 2.0; TB 1.7; TT 1.05 (estimated normal value: 38 sec).
INRs were calculated from the survey data using the equation INR=antilog(ISI.log R), where R is the ratio of abnormal plasma PT to local control PT (manual determinations only).

*values in parentheses give the number of participants.

LOELIGER: May I come back to the comments of Dr. Denson? Table 1 is taken from the French Etalonorme proficiency testing. If you translate the ratios as calculated into INRs for three rabbit thromboplastins using absorbed plasma, you get uniform INR values. The same is true for coumadinized plasmas. But if you use a different tissue type of thromboplastin, a large difference occurs: in that case the system with absorbed plasmas no longer works for normalization, whereas the system with coumadinized plasmas works well at an INR of 2.5 and reasonably well for clinical purposes at an INR of 3.5.

GRALNICK: What would your recommendation be concerning the INR? Should the in-house INR be established using normals and patients' data, or just patients' data? You showed data suggesting that there would be differences. The question is, what would you recommend, considering the fact that what we are looking for is the adequate control of patients on anticoagulant therapy?

VAN DEN BESSELAAR: If the data of normals and patients fit a single line, it is better to use that line. In that case the precision of the line is better than when we use patients' data alone. If there is a difference between the normals and the patients' line, then you should be careful, because the line for the combined data will introduce a bias in the INR values.

TOMENSON: Whatever method is used to calculate the INR, one must make use of normals. Otherwise one cannot make an estimate of the prothrombin time with 67/40 that corresponds to the mean normal time with your local reagent and hence cannot calculate an INR. The conversion formula of Dr. Van den Besselaar is not based on the patients' data alone since it makes implicit use of the distance of the normals from the patients' line.

LOELIGER: Another point is the question whether manufacturers producing lyophilized normal plasma should assign an INR value to the normal plasma. In Germany, a reference normal was established by means of a consensus-making mechanism (DIN 58939 Teil 1). A commercial normal plasma can deviate from the reference normal which can be expressed as a ratio, e.g. 0.9 or 1.1. Users of a thromboplastin and a commercial normal plasma should be informed about such a deviation from the reference normal.

I think that the commercial normal plasma should be calibrated, and the calibration value should be indicated on the label.

GEIGER: This is perfectly true if you want to use control plasmas for that purpose. We manufacture different thromboplastins, and there is no doubt that if you make a control, it will give quite different numbers with one thromboplastin as compared to the other one.

SPAETHE: Sometimes you have really very good comparisons between normals and anticoagulated patients. I now come back to my earlier question. When we as manufacturers calibrate against an internationally accepted thromboplastin, it is important that we calibrate like for like, i.e. PIVKA-sensitive versus PIVKA-sensitive and PIVKA-insensitive versus PIVKA-insensitive. When we do this, we have much better comparisons between normals and anticoagulated patients. All the manufacturers agree that we should standardize, but we must compare the right things.

LOELIGER: Dr. Spaethe is very much impressed by Prof. Hemker's work on PIVKAs. I am not sure whether the PIVKA effect is really so important for thromboplastin calibration. One of the manufacturers has a factor VII-insensitive thromboplastin which compares very well with all three BCR reference thromboplastins. I think that neither factor VII-insensitivity nor PIVKA-sensitivity of a thromboplastin interferes with calibration.

BERTINA: PIVKA-sensitivity in only one of the variables in the thromboplastins. If you are going to do this, you should have a completely separate procedure for standardization of each thromboplastin. I don't think that that is the purpose of standardization.

Chapter 9:   THE BRITISH SYSTEM OF ORAL ANTICOAGULANT CONTROL AND
ITS RELATION WITH THE WHO SYSTEM: CALIBRATION OF THE
PROPOSED SECOND WHO INTERNATIONAL REFERENCE THROMBO-
PLASTIN (BCT/253)

J.A. TOMENSON, J.M. THOMSON and L. POLLER

1. INTRODUCTION

Ingram (5) considered the evidence for instability of the
first International Reference Preparation (IRP) and suggested
that it was wise to replace this with a new preparation of human
brain made from British Comparative Thromboplastin (BCT). The
main reason for the latter was that the first IRP is designated
as a "combined" preparation i.e. containing adsorbed plasma as a
source of fibrinogen and is used with a different technique from
the Quick test where "plain" thromboplastins are utilised. The
use of the Quick prothrombin time test predominates on a world
basis for anticoagulant control whereas "combined" preparations
are used on a relatively limited scale (9). Reasons for the replacement of the primary IRP are summarised in Table 1. Furthermore, the requirement that the primary IRP be a "plain" Quick

Table 1. Reasons for replacement of first IRP.

---

1. Need for Quick test ("plain") primary IRP
2. Age and lack of stability studies on first IRP
3. Therapeutic considerations

---

test reagent receives further added impetus from the evidence put
forward at this meeting (15). This indicates that a major error
in calibration of thromboplastins arises from the use of 'unlike'
preparations. In this context the term 'unlike' preparations does
not refer to the species difference which was stressed in previous reports but to whether the thromboplastin is of "plain" or
"combined" type. The differences arising from the calibration of

reagents of different animal species are comparatively insignificant if these are both of the "plain" type.

The proposed hierarchical structure for calibration of thromboplastins is illustrated in Fig. 1. The replacement IRP preparation is related to the first human brain primary IRP and in turn to the secondary reference preparations of rabbit brain ("plain") and bovine brain ("combined").

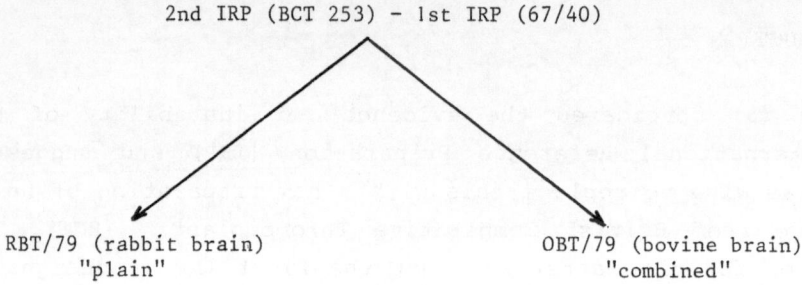

FIGURE 1. Proposed hierarchical structure for thromboplastin calibration

British Comparative Thromboplastin (BCT) has been widely used as a reference preparation for many years in many countries. Its application has largely been to assist in the preparation of national reference preparations and to calibrate manufacturers' commercial reagents. BCT is now well defined in therapeutic terms as it is prepared from a batch of Manchester Reagent which for many years has been used as the routine test reagent in the majority of UK hospitals. Table 2 details some of the published reports from overseas on the calibration of local or commercial preparations against BCT, illustrating the extent of its international application.

A batch of human brain thromboplastin produced in Manchester is therefore being submitted to WHO as a proposed second international reference preparation. An international collaborative exercise on calibration against the first IRP has been conducted at 17 centres, as well as accelerated degradation and on-going stability studies at the UK Reference Laboratory (14). The design and analysis of the international collaborative exercise undertaken to calibrate the proposed second WHO international reference thromboplastin (BCT/253) against the existing WHO IRP (67/40) are described later.

Table 2. Published correlations from overseas of BCT with other types of Quick test thromboplastin reagents

Bailey et al. (1971)	Canada
Bain et al. (1978)	Australia
Bradlow et al. (1974)	South Africa
Brink et al. (1976)	South Africa
Korsan-Bengtsen et al. (1977)	Sweden
Talalak (1979)	Thailand
Tankovski et al. (1977)	Bulgaria
Zucker et al. (1970)	USA

In Britain anticoagulant control is achieved through the large scale production of a Quick test thromboplastin with identical performance between successive batches. Each production lot of the routine reagent, Manchester Comparative Reagent (MCR), is matched against BCT to ensure identical sensitivity to the coumarin-induced defect. This standardisation procedure is discussed in Section 3 and results are given of the calibration of a batch of MCR against the IRP.

2. CALIBRATION OF THE PROPOSED SECOND WHO IRP

The design of this study was based on a European Economic Community, Bureau Communautaire de Référence (BCR) calibration exercise (10). Results were sought from eighteen designated centres (eight in the UK and ten overseas), approved by WHO. One of these, an overseas centre, failed to undertake the exercise. The number of participant laboratories compares favourably with the BCR study where the results from seven laboratories were considered sufficient to assess the effect of inter-laboratory variation.

2.1.Participants

2.1.1. Calibration of reference thromboplastin.

E.E. Mayne, Royal Victoria Hospital, Belfast, Great Britain

J.F. Davidson, Royal Infirmary, Glasgow, Great Britain

P. Barkhan, Guy's Hospital, London, Great Britain

J.W. Stewart, Middlesex Hospital, London, Great Britain

F.E. Preston, Hallamshire Hospital, Sheffield, Great Britain

R. Mibishan, King's College Hospital Medical School, London, Great Britain

P.B.A. Kernoff, Royal Free Hospital, London, Great Britain

L. Poller, UK Reference Laboratory for Anticoagulant Reagents and Control, Manchester, Great Britain

C. Carter, McMaster University, Hamilton, Canada

B. Bradlow, South African Institute for Medical Research, Johannesburg, South Africa

D.A. Triplett, Ball Memorial Hospital, Muncie, USA

P.M. Mannucci, Universita degli Studi di Milano, Italy

B.L. Evatt, Centres for Disease Control, Atlanta, USA

E.A. Loeliger, Interne Geneeskunde, Academisch Ziekenhuis, Leiden, The Netherlands

H. Beeser, University of Freiburg, German Federal Republic

K. Korsan-Bengtsen, Sahlgrenska Hospital, Goteberg, Sweden

K.A. Rickard, Royal Prince Alfred Hospital, Sydney, Australia

2.1.2. Statistical treatment of results.

J.A. Tomenson, UK Reference Laboratory for Anticoagulant Reagents and Control, Withington Hospital, Manchester, Great Britain

T.B.L. Kirkwood, National Institute for Medical Research, London, Great Britain

2.2 Experimental procedures

The protocol (Appendix 1) gives full details of the method of blood sample collection, equipment required and recommended procedures for patient selection, laboratory testing and recording of results. All reagents required for the laboratory testing were provided together with details of storage and/or reconstitution.

The principal features of the statistical design of the study are summarised below.

Each participating laboratory was asked to perform prothrombin time determinations on five different days if possible, to include the effect of daily variation. The testing each day was performed on four fresh normal and twelve coumarin plasmas. The coumarin plasmas were tested in the order in which they were collected with the normal plasmas always being the 1st, 8th, 9th and 16th plasmas to be tested in each session. Participant laboratories were asked to select patient samples displaying the widest possible levels of anticoagulation. The patients had to have been stabilised on oral anticoagulants for at least six weeks and give a prothrombin time ratio with the IRP of between 1.5 and 5.0.

2.3. Statistical Methodology

The statistical methodology used in this exercise was that developed for the calibration of thromboplastins which is described in a BCR report (10). In the BCR calibration exercise it was shown empirically that the logarithms of prothrombin times with different thromboplastins were approximately linearly related. In addition the linear relationship between the logarithms of prothrombin times displayed greater homoscedasticity than relationships between prothrombin times or ratios. The linear relationship between the logarithms of prothrombin times was estimated using a symmetric procedure which is referred to in the statistical literature as least squares estimation of a functional relationship (6) and described as orthogonal regression in the BCR study report. This symmetric estimation procedure allows for the fact that individual patients' prothrombin times determined using both thromboplastins show biological and experimental variation about the calibration line. The same strategy was adopted in this study using orthogonal regression to estimate the slope and intercept of the linear relationship between the logarithms of the prothrombin times with 67/40 and BCT/253. Estimates of the variability of the fitted calibration relationship, the standard deviation of regression, and the standard deviations of the slope and intercept were taken from Patefield (11).

For comparability with the BCR exercise, the data for a patient were only included for analysis if the prothrombin time with 67/40 was between 1.5 and 5.0 times the mean 67/40 prothrombin time of all normals of the same laboratory. Outliers were rejected on the basis of their orthogonal distance from the fitted calibration line. As in the BCR exercise an observation was considered to be outlying if its orthogonal distance was more than 3 times the standard deviation of regression (calculated with all points included). This criterion is directly analogous to that used for ordinary least squares regression.

In the BCR study an assumption was made that a single straight line describes the relationship between the logarithms of prothrombin times of both normals and patients and a test made for coincidence of the separate lines derived using only data from patients or normals. The assumption is important from the practical standpoint as it greatly simplifies the process of converting a prothrombin ratio from one thromboplastin to another. If the condition is met it can be shown (7) that

$$R_{67/40} = R_{BCT/253}^b$$

where $R_{67/40}$ and $R_{BCT/253}$ are the prothrombin time ratios for 67/40 and BCT/253 respectively, and b the slope of the calibration line. However, to achieve this parsimony of description it is only necessary to demonstrate that the mean logarithms of the prothrombin times of normals lie on the orthogonal regression line through patients' plasmas. Therefore in the present study only the simpler hypothesis was tested using an approximate test derived by Tomenson (15). A detailed examination, to be reported under Calibration Results, shows that the assumption was met at all but four centres.

The overall calibration was obtained by taking an unweighted average of the separate orthogonal regression lines calculated for the different centres. As a measure of inter-laboratory variation the standard deviations of the slope and intercept have been reported. These were calculated from the intercepts and slopes of the different laboratories. The calibration relationships of the different centres were also used to predict the prothrombin time with 67/40 corresponding to a prothrombin time with BCT/253 of 35 seconds which was approximately the average prothrombin time of patients in the study. The standard deviation of these predicted values is a more readily assimilated measure of the variation of the orthogonal regression line between laboratories.

2.4. Calibration Results

2.4.1. Exclusions. Table 3 gives the numbers of normal subjects and patients included in the study. The number of patients originally included in the study is shown as well as the number of exclusions due to a prothrombin time with 67/40 which was outside the given range. In addition eleven outlying pairs of observations were excluded according to the criterion of Section 2.3.

Table 3

Lab	Number of days	Number of normals	Number of patients	Number of exluded specimens below limits	above limits	outliers	Final total of plasmas
1	5	20	60	8	–	1	71
2	5	20	60	–	1	–	79
3	5	20	60	5	–	–	75
4	5	20	53	–	–	–	73
5	5	20	60	2	1	1	76
6	5	20	60	–	–	–	80
7	4	20	60	–	–	--	80
8	5	20	60	–	–	1	79
10	5	20	60	–	1	–	79
11	5	20	58	–	–	1	77
12	5	18	44	4	11	–	47
13	5	20	60	4	1	1	74
14	5	20	60	–	35	2	43
15	5	20	60	–	–	1	79
16	5	20	60	–	1	–	79
17	5	20	60	2	7	2	69
18	3	19	60	2	7	1	69

The outlying points were:

Lab 1	67/40 = 59.0 sec	BCT/253 = 28.0 sec
Lab 5	67/40 = 43.0 sec	BCT/253 = 42.0 sec
Lab 8	67/40 = 55.4 sec	BCT/253 = 24.2 sec
Lab 11	67/40 = 32.2 sec	BCT/253 = 30.4 sec
Lab 13	67/40 = 64.0 sec	BCT/253 = 30.0 sec
Lab 14	67/40 = 71.4 sec	BCT/253 =102.9 sec
	67/40 = 61.4 sec	BCT/253 = 71.4 sec
Lab 15	67/40 = 40.5 sec	BCT/253 = 35.0 sec
Lab 17	67/40 = 56.0 sec	BCT/253 = 51.0 sec
	67/40 = 52.5 sec	BCT/253 = 46.0 sec
Lab 18	67/40 = 65.0 sec	BCT/253 = 58.0 sec

Table 4a Means and standard deviations of the prothrombin times of the normal subjects

Lab	N	BCT/253		67/40	
		$\bar{x}$	s	$\bar{x}$	s
1	20	14.00	0.86	18.13	1.47
2	20	14.18	0.85	17.94	1.67
3	20	13.60	0.43	19.58	1.22
4	20	14.10	1.02	17.31	0.91
5	20	14.21	0.95	17.47	1.11
6	20	13.53	0.67	17.45	1.02
7	20	13.66	0.98	17.66	1.47
8	20	14.23	0.88	17.98	0.90
10	20	13.57	1.12	17.06	0.96
11	20	14.91	1.17	19.12	1.06
12	18	14.76	1.10	18.17	1.47
13	20	14.63	0.43	19.71	0.95
14	20	14.15	1.01	16.98	0.85
15	20	14.34	0.92	17.69	0.97
16	20	15.07	0.68	19.01	1.03
17	20	13.73	0.91	17.00	0.90
18	19	14.05	0.99	18.89	1.23

2.4.2. <u>Normal plasmas</u>. Table 4a summarises the data of normal subjects. Using both thromboplastins there were statistically significant differences between the mean normal prothrombin times for the 17 laboratories (one way analysis of variance, $p < 0.01$). The coefficient of variation of the normal prothrombin times averaged over the seventeen laboratories was 6.2% for both BCT/253 and 67/40. These results suggest that the two reference preparations are very similar in terms of their inter-ampoule variability as the other components of the coefficient of variation will not differ between thromboplastins.

2.4.3. Patient plasmas. The complete set of patient plasmas submitted for analysis is a further indication of the variability in the intensity of anticoagulation in different countries. The highest mean prothrombin ratios were obtained by the two United States centres and the one Australian centre. A mean ratio of 6.1 with 67/40 at one of these centres necessitated the exclusion of thirty-five of the sixty patient results. At the other extreme eight exclusions of inadequately dosed patients were required at one UK centre where the mean ratio with 67/40 was 1.9.

The means and standard deviations of the prothrombin times of the patients remaining after exclusions had been made are shown in Table 4b. There was still a considerable variation between laboratories in the distributions of patient plasmas included in the analysis.

Table 4b Means and standard deviations of the prothrombin times of the patients included in the analysis

Lab	N	BCT/253		67/40	
		$\bar{x}$	s	$\bar{x}$	s
1	51	26.98	4.33	36.21	6.16
2	59	34.34	9.62	48.63	13.55
3	55	36.39	8.03	51.33	10.02
4	53	32.05	6.44	44.00	8.96
5	56	38.18	10.36	48.16	13.00
6	60	36.70	8.06	51.84	12.66
7	60	33.58	6.75	46.13	8.84
8	59	37.88	10.00	54.41	14.28
10	59	36.16	8.17	50.34	11.76
11	57	32.27	7.95	44.28	10.83
12	29	44.90	12.70	60.04	16.80
13	54	31.66	6.15	47.36	10.28
14	25	49.99	10.47	65.77	12.11
15	59	37.43	9.21	52.40	13.29
16	59	32.33	5.79	48.18	9.18
17	49	34.23	8.26	48.80	12.38
18	50	40.74	13.12	56.51	17.21

2.4.4. Orthogonal regression of BCT/253 against 67/40. Table 5 gives the equations of the orthogonal regression lines for the different laboratories. The standard deviations of the slope and intercept and the standard deviation about the regression line are also given. Also shown in Table 5 are estimated prothrombin times with 67/40 corresponding to the mean patient prothrombin time with BCT/253 of 35 seconds. These predicted values were determined using the orthogonal regression lines of each laboratory. Figures showing all the data points included for analysis together with the fitted lines can be found in Appendix 2. The reported lines are based on the combined data from patients and normals. The decision to use the line through patients and normals was made after testing the hypothesis that the mean logarithm of the normal prothrombin times for each thromboplastin lay on the orthogonal regression line derived from patients' data for each laboratory. This hypothesis was statistically rejected at four centres, laboratories 8, 14, 15, 16 ($p < 0.01$). It should also be noted that the mean logarithms of the normal prothrombin times lie below the orthogonal regression line of the patients at 15 of the 17 centres. This suggests a small degree of curvilinearity in the overall calibration relationship. However, laboratories 14 and 16 display the most significant differences but in each case graphical inspection of the data shows that the overall orthogonal regression line describes the patients' data adequately. For this reason it was felt appropriate to use the line through patients and normals for all laboratories.

Visual inspection of the data shows that a linear relationship between the logarithms of prothrombin times is a good description of the data from all laboratories. Good homoscedasticity has also been achieved in most cases by the use of logarithms. The good fit of the calibration model is apparent in the low standard deviations around the regression lines shown in Table 5. The complete set of regression lines is shown in Figure 2. The slopes of the orthogonal regression lines range from 0.973 to 1.195 but over the therapeutic range the majority of lines intersect and run close together. Some of this variability might have been due to the large differences in the prothrombin times of patients included by different laboratories. In fitting the orthogonal regression line the sample distribution of patient plasmas is

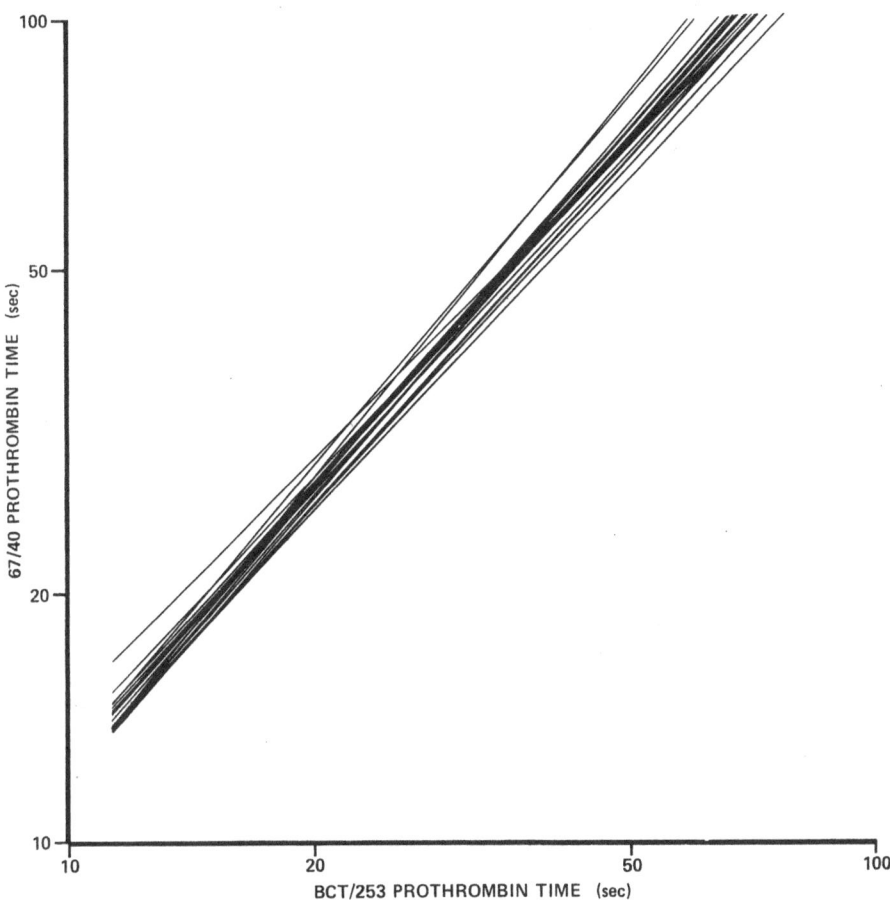

FIGURE 2. The orthogonal regression lines y = a + bx for each of the seventeen laboratories. x and y are prothrombin time/s on a logarithmic scale using thromboplastins BCT/253 and 67/40 respectively.

particularly important as regards the precision of estimates of the slope and intercept and the representativeness of these estimates. However, there does not appear to be any noticeable relationship between the sampling distribution of patient plasmas as shown in Table 4b and the orthogonal regression lines given in Table 5.

Table 5   Orthogonal regression equations $y = a + bx$ for BCT/253 (x-axis) versus 67/40 (y-axis). x and y are in log PT/sec. Tabulated are intercept a, standard deviation of the intercept s(a), slope b, standard deviation of the slope s(b) and the standard deviation about the orthogonal regression line s. P is the predicted 67/40 prothrombin time corresponding to a 35 sec prothrombin time with BCT/253

Lab	N	a	s(a)	b	s(b)	s	P (sec)
1	71	0.046	0.035	1.057	0.026	0.021	47.7
2	79	-0.016	0.029	1.108	0.020	0.022	49.5
3	75	0.192	0.022	0.973	0.015	0.019	49.5
4	73	-0.045	0.036	1.120	0.025	0.024	48.4
5	76	0.060	0.022	1.026	0.015	0.019	44.0
6	80	0.001	0.025	1.095	0.017	0.021	49.2
7	80	0.050	0.023	1.057	0.016	0.018	48.1
8	79	-0.014	0.025	1.108	0.017	0.021	49.8
10	79	0.005	0.031	1.088	0.021	0.025	48.4
11	77	0.035	0.032	1.067	0.022	0.022	48.1
12	47	0.012	0.038	1.069	0.026	0.030	45.9
13	74	-0.032	0.030	1.138	0.021	0.020	53.1
14	43	0.009	0.026	1.065	0.018	0.022	45.0
15	79	-0.035	0.019	1.114	0.013	0.015	48.4
16	79	-0.123	0.025	1.195	0.017	0.015	52.7
17	69	-0.054	0.025	1.135	0.018	0.019	50.0
18	69	0.115	0.021	1.017	0.014	0.018	48.5

The calibration protocol stipulated that the coagulation endpoint should be determined manually wherever possible but if a coagulometer was used both tests must be carried out on the same instrument. However, one centre used a Fibrometer for BCT/253 and a Coagulation Profiler for 67/40. For this reason it was felt that the results of this centre, laboratory 12, should not be used to determine the overall calibration relationship even though their results showed agreement with those of other centres.

The results of the remaining sixteen laboratories were combined by taking the unweighted mean of the intercepts and slopes. These are shown in Table 6 together with measures of variability of the slopes and intercepts among the sixteen laboratories. It is worth noting that a calibrated value of 1.087 would have been obtained had all patient plasmas apart from outliers been included in the analysis. However, it would be unwise to infer that the calibration could be used outside the specified range as only one laboratory has a substantial number of observations outside the range. The variability between laboratories of the predicted 67/40 prothrombin time corresponding to the mean patient prothrombin time with BCT/253 is also given. The standard deviation is only 2.3 seconds which demonstrates the closeness of the orthogonal regression lines in the middle range of oral anticoagulation dosage according to the British system for anticoagulant control.

Table 6 Unweighted means of the orthogonal regression line y = a + bx for BCT/253 versus 67/40 and P the predicted 67/40 prothrombin time corresponding to a 35 sec prothrombin time with BCT/253. x and y are in log time/sec. S_a, S_b and S_p are the standard deviation of the intercepts, slopes and predicted values of the different laboratories.

intercept a	slope b	predicted value P (sec)	between laboratory variation S_a	S_b	S_p
0.012	1.085	48.78	0.073	0.054	2.27

3. STANDARDISATION AND CALIBRATION OF MANCHESTER REAGENT

3.1. Standardisation

The success of MCR production depends on the ability of the manufacturer to reproduce exactly the performance characteristics of previous batches. Recently the new BCR calibration has been adopted to further ensure that within the limits of statistical error, the sensitivity of batches remains constant. However,

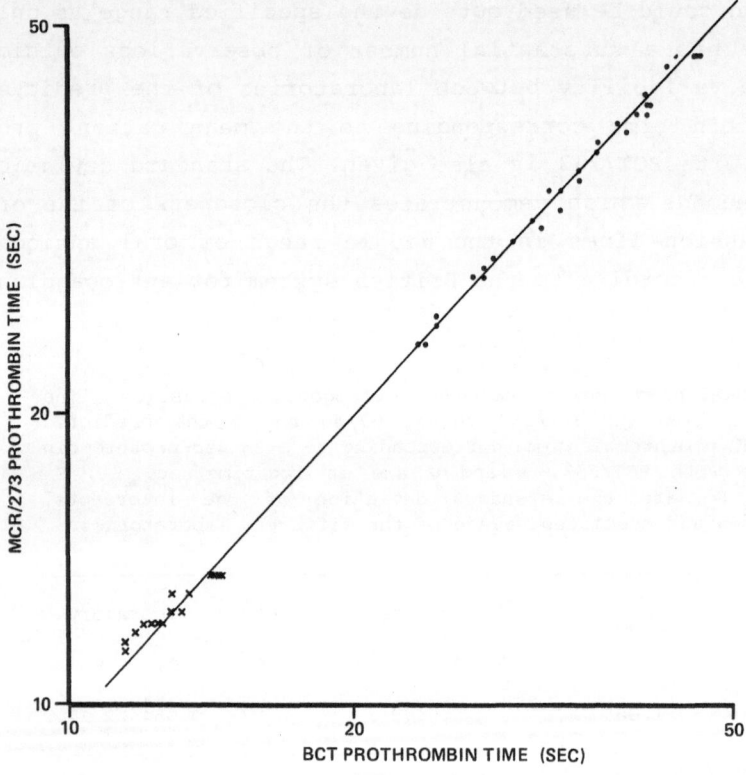

FIGURE 3. Data on log (time/s) scale of patients and normals obtained with BCT (x-axis) versus those obtained with MCR/273 (y-axis).

calibration constitutes only one procedure used to confirm that each new batch gives identical results to previous batches. Only the calibration of successive batches will be considered here.

Each new batch of MCR emerges as the best of several trial batches through a process of adjustment by dilution and/or recombination. To confirm that its sensitivity matches that of previous batches it is calibrated against BCT and the two preceding batches of MCR. In this respect BCT acts as a house standard and it is worth noting that its sensitivity will have been monitored by at least three external centres. An example of a calibration against BCT is given in Fig. 3. It can be seen that the standard deviation about the calibration line is extremely low. The average size of this standard deviation is 0.007 which is considerably less than that observed in the BCR study or the international collaborative exercise. For this reason it is possible to achieve a high degree of precision using a much smaller number of plasmas than the 60 patients and 20 normals recommended in the BCR protocol. Calibration is in fact performed using 12 patients' plasmas and the plasmas of six normal controls. Even using this number of plasmas it is possible to estimate the slope of the calibration line with greater precision than that achieved by any laboratory in the international collaborative exercise. Over a two-month period, the recommended shelf life of MCR, a total of four such calibrations are performed on each batch. This ensures that a detailed retrospective assessment of the production process can be made and provides evidence of the stability of each batch of the reagent.

The success of the procedure can be seen in the sensitivity of the three successive batches of MCR shown in Table 7. The sensitivity is expressed as an International Sensitivity Index (ISI) which is the slope of the calibration line if compared with the IRP. The standard deviations about the calibration line shown in the Table are those obtained in the calibration against BCT. It can be seen that the maximum change in sensitivity from the mean of the three batches is less than 1%. It is clearly unnecessary to issue an ISI for each batch since for all practical purposes

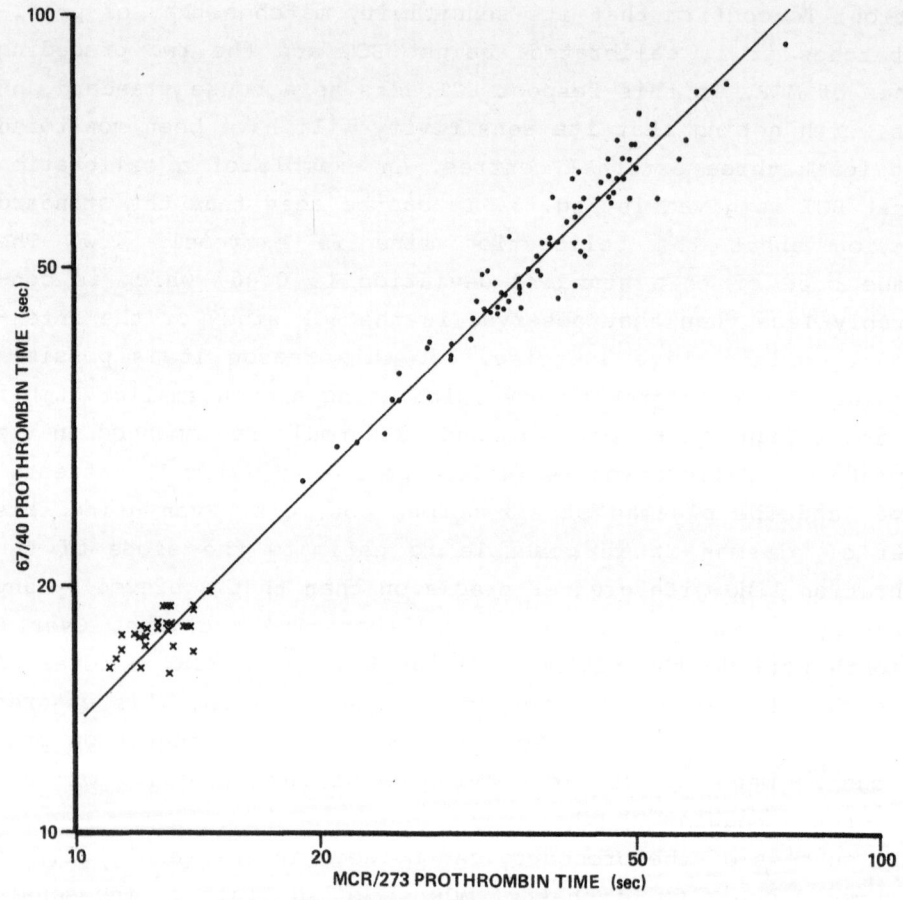

FIGURE 4. Data on log (time/s) scale of patients and normals obtained with MCR/273 (x-axis) versus those obtained with the IRP 67/40 (y-axis).

they are identical. This is a highly satisfactory situation for the user as it avoids the necessity to convert prothrombin ratios.

Table 7   ISIs of three successive batches of MCR

	Batch no.			Mean of three batches
	272	273	274	
ISI	0.996	0.990*	0.985	0.995
Standard deviation around calibration line (against BCT)	0.008	0.007	0.007	–

*estimated from a direct calibration against the IRP (67/40)

3.2 Calibration

Periodic calibration will in future be made against he proposed second IRP to eliminate the possibility of a drift in the sensitivity of the Manchester reagent. A calibration was recently performed for batch no. 273 against the present IRP. The calibration was performed according to the protocol of the international exercise and two further days of testing came from a separate exercise performed concurrently. A total of 83 patients' plasmas and 28 plasmas from normal controls were included and the ISI was calculated to be 0.990. Figure 4 shows the data from this exercise together with the orthogonal regression line. Additional confirmation of the sensitivity of MCR was provided by a separate calibration against BCT/099, the BCR human reference thromboplastin. In this exercise the slope of the calibration line was found to be 0.948 which taken with the known ISI of BCT/099, 1.048, gave an estimated ISI of 0.994.

REFERENCES

1.   Bailey EI, Harper TA, Pinkertin PH. The "therapeutic range" of the one-stage prothrombin time in the control of anticoagulant therapy: the effect of different thromboplastin preparations. Canad Med Ass J 1971; 105: 1041-1044.

2. Bain B, Forster T, Sleigh B. Control of oral anticoagulants by the prothrombin time: a plea for uniformity. Aust Med J 1978; 2: 459-461.
3. Bradlow BA, Saunder C, Whitbread P et al. Standardisation of the laboratory control of anticoagulant therapy. SA Med J 1974; 48: 1857-1862.
4. Brink S, Cloete H, Roberts R, Holm W. Laboratoriumstandaardisasie en kwaliteitscontrole in antistolterapie. SA Med J 1976; 50: 205-208.
5. Ingram GIC. The stability of the WHO reference thromboplastin NIBS&C 67/40. Thromb Haemostas 1979; 42: 1135-1140.
6. Kendall MG, Stuart A. The advanced theory of statistics, Vol. 2, Chapter 29. Charles Griffin, London. 1961.
7. Kirkwood TBL. Calibration of reference thromboplastins and standardisation of the prothrombin time ratio. Thromb Haemostas 1983; 49: 238-244.
8. Korsan-Bengtsen K, Johsen M, Pehrsson NG. Comparison between British Comparative Thromboplastin (BCT) and a factor II - VII - X determination method (Simplastin A) based on fresh plasma samples from dicoumarol-treated patients. Thromb Haemostas 1977; 37: 98-103.
9. Lam-Po Tang PRLC, Poller L. Oral anticoagulant therapy and its control: an international survey. Thromb Diathes Haemorrh 1975; 34: 419-425.
10. Loeliger EA, Van den Besselaar AMHP, Hermans J, Van der Velde EA. Certification of three reference materials for thromboplastins. BCR Information. Commission of the European Communities, Brussels. 1981
11. Patefield WM. On the information matrix in the linear functional relationship problem. Applied Statistics 1977; 26: 69.
12. Talalak P. Current oral anticoagulant practice and its laboratory control in Thailand: II. Comparison of rabbit brain and human brain thromboplastin, calibration against standard reference thromboplastin. J Med Ass Thailand 1979; 62: 618-629.
13. Tankovski I, Lisichkov T, Angelova Tsv, Buchvarova V. Study of the standardized Bulgarian thromboplastin for prothrombin time determination. Savr Med 1977; 28: 40-43.
14. Thomson JM, Stevenson KJ, Tomenson JA. Report on proposed second WHO international reference thromboplastin, human, plain, to replace the WHO international reference preparation, human, combined. Submitted to WHO. 1983.
15. Tomenson JA. A statistician's independent evaluation. This volume, Chapter 5.
16. Zucker S, Brosious E, Cooper GR. One-stage prothrombin time survey. Am J Clin Pathol 1970; 53: 340-347.

APPENDIX 1: Protocol of calibration of proposed second WHO international reference thromboplastin (BCT/253) against existing primary WHO International Reference Preparation (67/40)

A.1. Experimental design

Testing should be done on five separate days, which need not be consecutive. On each one of these days obtain: freshly prepared plasma samples from four normal individuals and twelve patients. A one-day experiment should be completed within four hours from the collection of the blood. The time schedule of a one-day experiment is as follows:

1.

First 1-2 hours: collection of blood and preparation of thromboplastin suspension. The blood should be drawn from four normal subjects (see A.2.1) and twelve patients stabilised on oral anticoagulants (see A.2.2.). Centrifuge blood immediately after withdrawal and transfer the plasma into a non-wettable, stoppered container. Maintain at room temperature until required for testing. (See A.3.1.-A.3.4.)

2.

Second 2 hours: testing of the sixteen plasma samples with the two thromboplastins according to the design described in section A.6.

Note: a) Single, not duplicate determinations should be performed.

b) The two determinations on each plasma (one with each thromboplastin) should be performed immediately after each other. Thus the two determinations on an individual plasma should be completed before starting the next subject's plasma. This order of testing means that timing of the determinations will be linked together as closely as possible. The order of testing is indicated by Roman numerals in the scheme given under A.6.

c) The order in which the patients are tested shall preferably be the same as the order of collection. The first
normal control sample should be collected before the
coumarin-treated patients' samples and the fourth normal
control collected last, after the patients' samples.

A.2. Selection of normals and patients

A.2.1. <u>Normals</u>. The normal subjects must be ambulant a-
dults. If possible, for a one-day experiment, include two males
and two females. Select different normals on each day of testing.

A.2.2 <u>Patients</u>. The patients should have been stabilised on
oral anticoagulants for at least six weeks. Participant centres
are requested to select the patient samples displaying the widest
possible variety of levels of anticoagulation, which, for most of
the commercially available rabbit thromboplastins, represents
prothrombin time ratios from 1.2 to 2.2. times normal and for
British Comparative Thromboplastin ratios from 1.5-5.0 (this
range approximates to 1.5-5 in terms of WHO reference thromboplastin, preparation 67/40).

A.3. Sample collection

A.3.1. The specimen shall be collected, by clean venipunc-
ture, into 1/10 volume of sterile trisodium citrate 0.109 mol/l;
blood shall preferably be drawn with plastic or silicone-coated
syringe and transferred into a plastic or silicone-coated container. If an evacuated tube is employed the brand selected must
be sufficiently siliconised (see section A.5.2.).

A.3.2. The blood shall be centrifuged immediately after
collection (approx. 800 g = approx. 2500 rpm) for 5 min, at room
temperature.

A.3.3. The plasma shall be transferred by siliconised or
plastic pipette to a stoppered, non-wettable container.

A.3.4. The stoppered vessel containing the plasma is kept at room temperature until testing.

NOTE: a minimum of 0.5 ml per plasma specimen must be available.

A.4. Thromboplastins (BCT/253 and 67/40)

A.4.1. Upon arrival the two thromboplastins should be stored at -20°C until required.

NOTE: The reconstitution fluid (phenolised water: 250 mg/l) for BCT/253 and the 3.2 mmol/l $CaCl_2$ for reconstitution of 67/40 should be stored at +4°C.

A.4.2. For BCT/253 reconstitute each ampoule with 0.5 ml phenolised water. Leave thromboplastin in ampoule. Keep at room temperature.

A.4.3. For 67/40 reconstitute each ampoule with 2.0 ml of 3.2 mmol/l $CaCl_2$. Leave thromboplastin in ampoule. Keep at room temperature.

A.4.4. Ampoules of thromboplastin BCT/253 and 67/40 should be opened as follows: Make a deep scratch round the ampoule with a glass file provided (on the 'neck' of BCT/253 ampoules) and then break off the top of the ampoule manually. This should be done under cover of a cloth as a protection against splintering of the glass and exposure of rough edges. Extreme caution should be observed during the opening to avoid loss of contents.

A.4.5. If difficulty is experienced in opening the ampoules by the method described in section A.4.4., the following alternative can be adopted: Scratch the 'neck' of the ampoule of BCT/253 or the ampoule of 67/40 with the glass file provided. The scratch should be sufficient to make a deep indentation. Touch the ampoule at this point with a heated glass rod in order to break the glass. Warning is given that excess heat may be deleterious to the thromboplastin. Open the ampoule by carefully removing the portion of glass above the break.

A.4.6. Ensure that the thromboplastin is completely resuspended before use. Gentle tapping on the side of the ampoule with a finger will facilitate resuspension. It is not necessary or desirable to shake the suspension vigorously.

A.4.7. Four ampoules of BCT/253 and four ampoules of 67/40 should be sufficient for one day's exercise, i.e. the testing of sixteen plasmas, using single determinations.

A.5. Other reagents and equipment

A.5.1. Sodium citrate 0.109 mol/l; for blood collection.
$CaCl_2$ 25 mmol/l; for recalcification of plasma/thromboplastin mixture, using BCT/253 (provided)
Store at 4°C.

NOTE: Use fresh aliquots of the above reagent each day.

GENERAL NOTE: Do not use thromboplastin which has been reconstituted for longer than two hours.

A.5.2. Equipment. All equipment, including syringes and evacuated tubes, must be silicone-coated (many of the commercially available vacuum systems for blood collection are insufficiently siliconised) or made of good quality plastic material to prevent contact activation of coagulation factors.

Plastic or siliconised syringes and/or containers for blood collection.

Plastic or siliconised containers with suitable caps or covered with parafilm (do not use rubber stoppers) for storage of blood or plasma.

Plastic or siliconised pipettes for transfer of plasma from (centrifuged) blood tubes into containers for storage of plasma.

Plastic or siliconised pipettes for transfer of plasma into glass test tubes at the time of testing.

Use non-siliconised disposable glass test tubes for the actual testing.

Thermostat ("water-bath") with water temperature of 37°C (tolerance limits: 37.0°C±0.2°C).

Use calibrated thermometer.

A.6. Testing procedure

Pipettes, test tubes, dispensers and thermostats customarily used in the laboratory must fulfil all of the above mentioned preconditions. For plasma, all new pipetting tips must be used for each test.

The sequence of testing is indicated in the following scheme by Roman numerals:

Sample	BCT/253	67/40
normal 1	I	II
patient 1	III	IV
patient 2	V	VI
patient 3	VII	VIII
patient 4	IX	X
patient 5	XI	XII
patient 6	XIII	XIV
normal 2	XV	XVI
normal 3	XVII	XVIII
patient 7	XIX	XX
patient 8	XXI	XXII
patient 9	XXIII	XXIV
patient 10	XXV	XXVI
patient 11	XXVII	XXVIII
patient 12	XXIX	XXX
normal 4	XXXI	XXXII

The coagulation endpoint should be determined manually (tilt-tube technique) wherever possible. Test tubes should be kept under water at 37°C as much as possible in order to maintain optimal temperature. The use of an illuminated water-bath avoids the necessity for removal of the tube from the water during tilting. If you have to use a coagulometer both tests must be carried out on the same instrument, adjusting for the different delivery volumes of the two thromboplastin reagents.

Proceed as follows: Place two glass test tubes in the water-bath for testing according to the order indicated in Roman numerals in the scheme under A.6.

For 67/40: a) transfer 0.4 ml thromboplastin to the test tube; b) incubate for 2 min; c) add 0.05 ml plasma to the test tube, mix and start the stopwatch immediately; d) tilt test-tube manually according to technique described above. Record clotting time (sec).

For BCT/253 not containing calcium: a) transfer 0.1 ml thromboplastin to the test tube; b) incubate for 2 min; c) add 0.1 ml plasma; d) mix gently with the thromboplastin; e) wait 1 min for incubation to reach the optimal reaction temperature; f) recalcify with 0.1 ml prewarmed $CaCl_2$ 25 mmol/l; g) tilt test-tube manually according to technique described above. Record clotting time (sec).

APPENDIX 2

<u>Scattergrams of prothrombin time/s on a logarithmic scale with orthogonal regression lines</u>

FIGURE A2: Data on a log (time/s) scale of patients and normals obtained with BCT/253 (x-axis) versus those obtained with 67/40 (y-axis). The orthogonal regression line is drawn and only data accepted for analysis are shown.
For laboratories 14 and 16 the orthogonal regression line for patients only is also shown as a broken line.

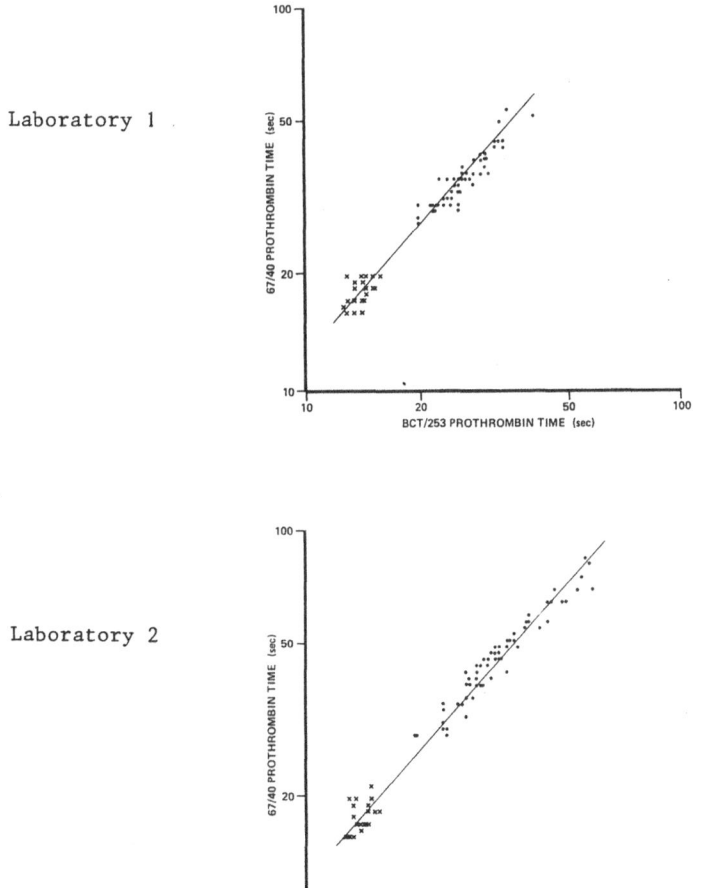

Laboratory 1

Laboratory 2

190

Laboratory 3

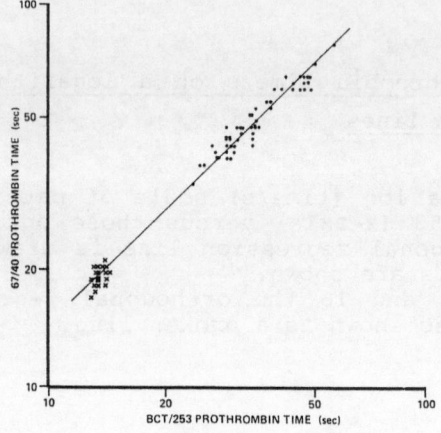

Laboratory 4

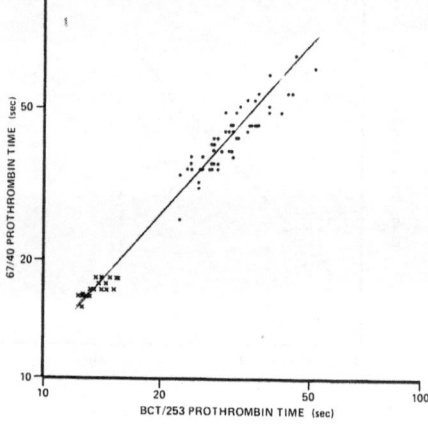

Laboratory 5

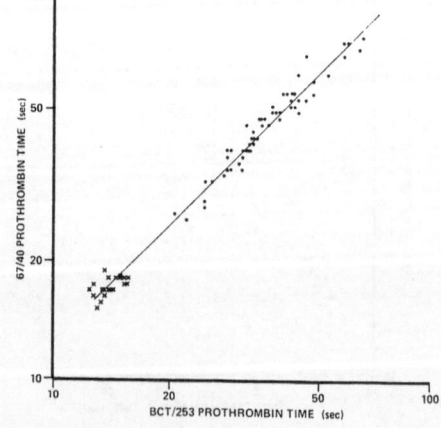

Laboratory 6

Laboratory 7

Laboratory 8

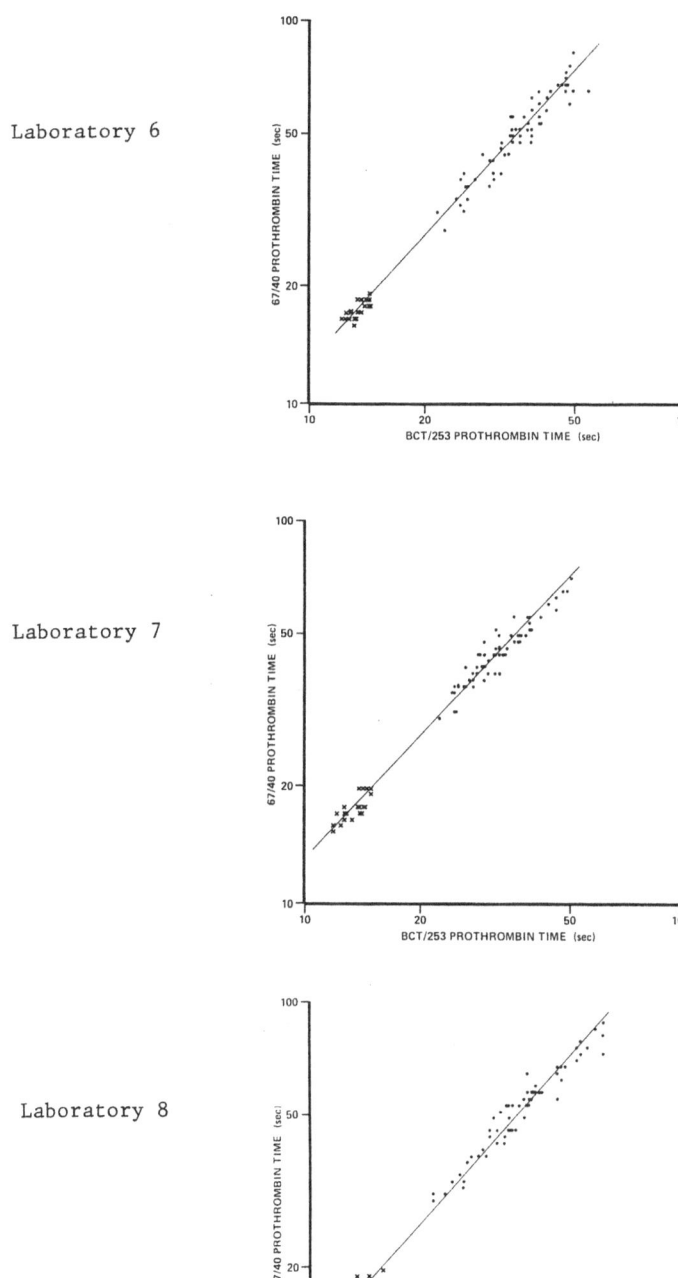

Laboratory 10

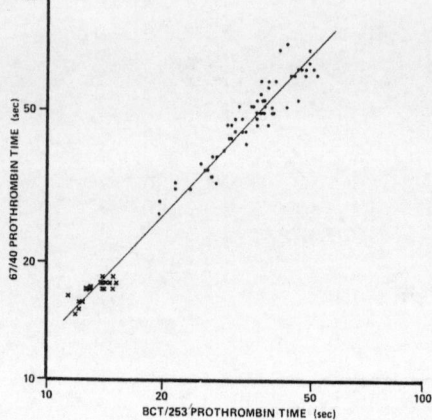

Laboratory 11

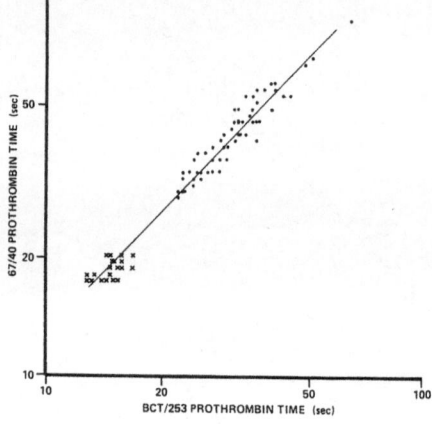

Laboratory 12

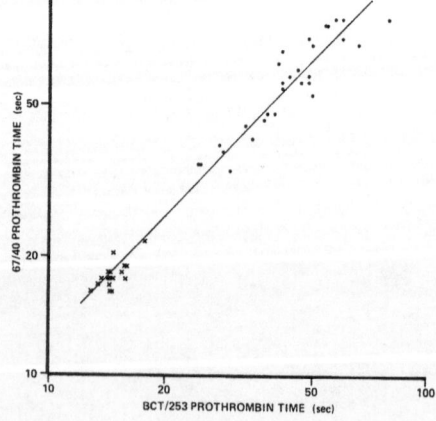

Laboratory 13

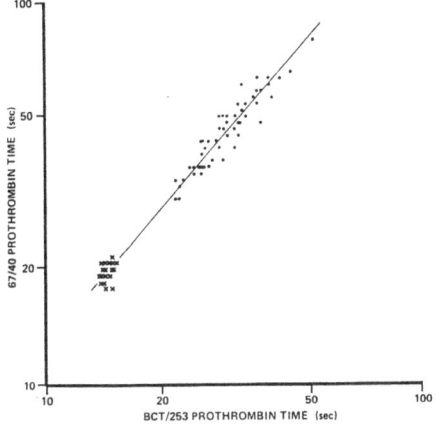

Laboratory 14

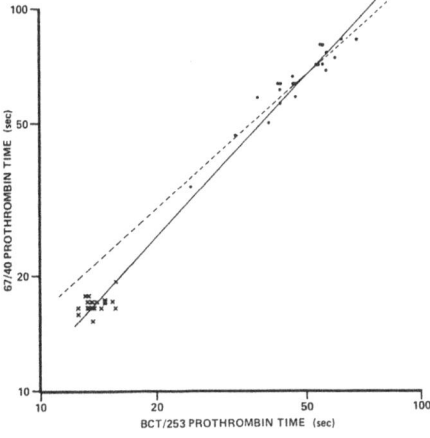

Laboratory 15

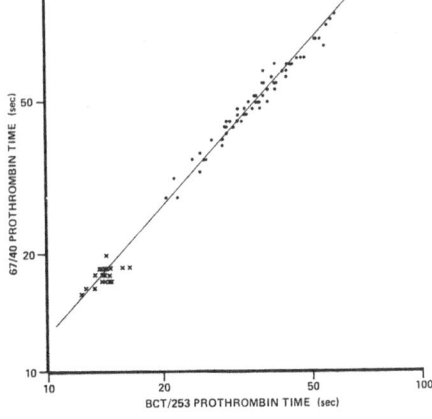

Laboratory 16

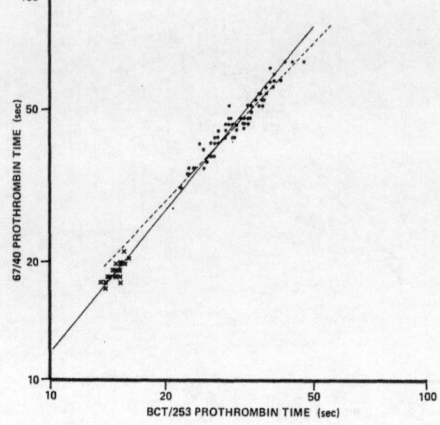

Laboratory 17

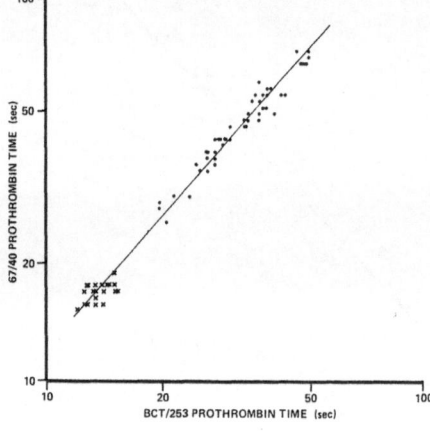

Laboratory 18

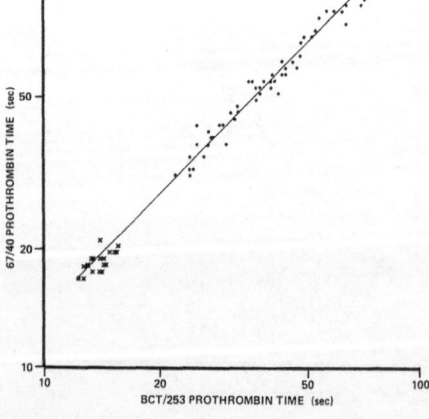

Chapter 10:   ANOMALIES OF THROMBOPLASTIN NOMENCLATURE

B.McD. DUXBURY

We are approaching the International STANDARDISATION of THROMBOPLASTINS and the establishment of an International PRO-THROMBIN TIME RATIO.

There are, however, some anomalies of Thromboplastin NOMEN-CLATURE and I feel that these should be considered now, so that if a change is required this can be published together with the report of this meeting (Table I). We can only suggest a change - the decision would have to be made after careful consideration by the British and International Standardisation Committees.

The first anomaly is Manchester Comparative Reagent (M.C.R.) for the inclusion of 'Comparative' in the title falsely implies that the reagent can be used for Calibration - but it is only a 'calibrated' reagent. This is used by the majority of hospitals in the U.K. and in recognition should have a NATIONAL and not a Regional designation. The title of the reagent should be speci-fic and so THROMBOPLASTIN should be included. When using M.C.R. the Prothrombin Time is reported as the BRITISH RATIO - which is illogical and misleading. I therefore suggest a change to BRITISH THROMBOPLASTIN with a logical BRITISH RATIO.

The other suggested change of nomenclature is more contro-versial, but I feel that it should be considered at the same time. The term 'Comparative' is now historical and is only a British term. It has served its purpose and should be replaced by an International Nomenclature.

In line with the 'Reference Materials' proposed by the Euro-pean Community Bureau of Reference, it is suggested that British Comparative Thromboplastin (B.C.T.) be re-designated BRITISH REFERENCE THROMBOPLASTIN. In his early publications, Dr. Poller states 'The result with B.C.T. is termed the British CORRECTED Ratio'. Since these early publications, many have adopted 'Comparative' but this is technically incorrect for such a change can only be made by a further publication and there has been none to date. However, this argument of nomenclature could be conveniently settled by the rapid introduction of the INTERNATIONAL NORMALISED RATIO.

Table 1.   Anomalies of thromboplastin nomenclature

PRESENT DESIGNATION	REASON FOR SUGGESTED CHANGE	SUGGESTED CHANGE	RATIO DESIGNATION
M.C.R.	1. Reagent is used Nationally and Designation should be NATIONAL and NOT Regional	B.T. BRITISH THROMBOPLASTIN (Phenolised Calibrated Reagent)	B.R. BRITISH RATIO
	2. 'Comparative' FALSELY implies that REAGENT can be used for Calibration (i.e. is a 'Standard' or a 'Reference' Reagent)		
	3. THROMBOPLASTIN should be in the title		
	4. Prothrombin Time with Reagent (M.C.R.) is reported as BRITISH RATIO (B.R.)		
B.C.T.	1. COMPARATIVE is now 'historical'	B.R.T.	B.C.R.
	2. Material is a 'REFERENCE MATERIAL' and should be named as such	BRITISH REFERENCE THROMBOPLASTIN (Lyophilised Secondary Standard) B.R.T. (253) (European Primary Standard - I.R.P.)	British Corrected ratio BUT PHASED-OUT with the introduction of I.N.R.

CHAPTER 11:   COMPARISON OF A HIGHLY SENSITIVE RABBIT BRAIN THROMBOPLASTIN, DADE THROMBOPLASTIN FS, WITH A HUMAN BRAIN THROMBOPLASTIN, MANCHESTER COMPARATIVE THROMBOPLASTIN

R. SPAETHE and I. SHIRLEY

1. INTRODUCTION

A few years ago, a field trial was carried out in which a large number of plasma samples (100 normals, 806 anticoagulated patients, as well as patients with deficiencies of the factors II, V, VII and X) were tested with a newly developed rabbit brain thromboplastin (Thromboplastin FS) and with Human Brain Thromboplastin prepared by Prof. Duckert in Basel (1). Both reagents behaved similarly over the whole range of measurement (fig. 1). The "calibration constant" (according to the concept of Biggs and Denson) of Thromboplastin FS relative to Human Brain Thromboplastin Basel was determined with 0.986.

In this contribution we assess the sensitivity of Thromboplastin FS to single coagulation factor deficiencies and to dilutions of normal plasma. Furthermore, we compare Thromboplastin FS with another human brain thromboplastin, Manchester Comparative Thromboplastin, in a study of 230 patients under oral anticoagulant treatment.

2. METHODS

2.1. Thromboplastins

Dade Thromboplastin FS is an acetone-dehydrated rabbit brain thromboplastin.

Manchester Comparative Thromboplastin (MCT) is a saline extract of human brain provided by the National Reference Laboratory for Anticoagulant Reagents and Control at Manchester, UK.

2.2. Techniques and Patients

Prothrombin times of 230 long-term stably anticoagulated patients were determined by manual tilt tube technique. The patients were treated according to the regimen of MCT.

2.3. Statistical analysis

The statistical analysis of comparison was done by a linear regression procedure $y = a + b x$ and by power function $y = a x^b$ ($a > o$). Ordinary regression techniques have the basic assumption that the deviations of the observed points from the true relationship are solely due to random fluctuations present in the measurements of one of the two variables. This is an unrealistic assumption.

A different statistical procedure (2) is more appropriate. This technique regards both methods of analysis as equivalent and a normal distribution of the values compared is not an assumption.

3. RESULTS

3.1 Factor sensitivity: Comparison Thromboplastin FS - Human Brain Thromboplastin Basel - British Comparative Thromboplastin

In Table 1 we show the coagulation factor sensitivity of two human brain preparations in comparison with the rabbit brain preparation. We looked at the ratio (deficiency plasma in sec./ fresh normal pool (FNP) in sec.) in substrate plasmas from patients with hereditary coagulation factor deficiency. Human Brain Thromboplastin Basel and Thromboplastin FS have nearly the same sensitivity. BCT was less sensitive. From these results we could expect that normals, factor deficient patients and patients under oral anticoagulation should give us comparable prothrombin times as demonstrated for FS and Human Brain Thromboplastin Basel (fig. 1).

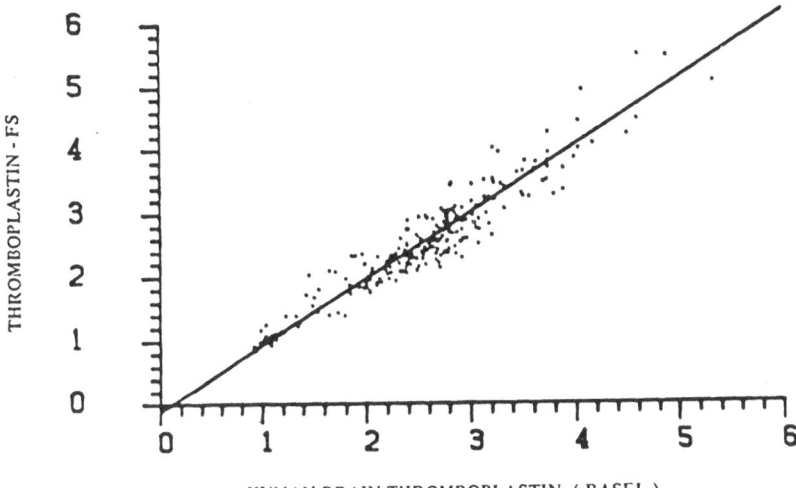

FIGURE 1: Comparison of prothrombin time ratios for Thromboplastin FS (y-axis) with ratios for human brain thromboplastin Basel (x-axis). Data are shown of 30 normals, 19 liver patients and 200 patients treated with oral anticoagulants. Measurements were performed by Prof. Duckert's laboratory (Basel). The regression line for all data is shown.

Table 1   Sensitivity of thromboplastins to coagulation factors. Prothrombin times were determined in substrate plasmas from patients with hereditary coagulation factor deficiencies and in fresh normal plasma. The ratio patient/normal is given.

Factor	BCT	FS	human brain Basel
X	5.6	7.4	7.0
VII	4.5	6.0	6.7
V	2.4	6.0	5.7
II	4.2	8.1	4.0

3.2. Comparison Thromboplastin FS - Manchester Comparative Thromboplastin (MCT)

3.2.1. Calibration curve. We established with dilutions of a normal plasma pool (CoagCal^R) in saline a calibration curve for the prothrombin times of MCT and FS (fig. 2). CoagCal^R, a lyoph-ilized normal pool of more than 100 donors, has been calibrated against a deep frozen (-70°C) normal pool from more than 100 donors. CoagCal^R was previously shown to be a good calibrator for all coagulation tests (3).

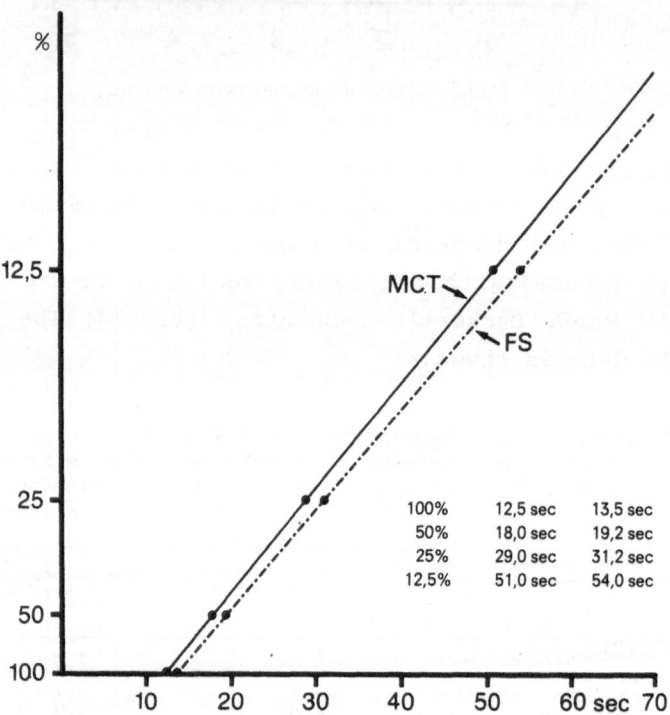

Comparison MCT / Dade FS
dilution curve: CoagCal® (Merz + Dade) as normal pool
diluted with physiol. NaCl
manual tilt technique

100%	12,5 sec	13,5 sec
50%	18,0 sec	19,2 sec
25%	29,0 sec	31,2 sec
12,5%	51,0 sec	54,0 sec

FIGURE 2: Prothrombin time (x-axis) as a function of normal plasma dilution in 0.9% NaCl expressed as percentage (y-axis).

Calculations of the slope of the curves show a similar behav-iour of FS and MCT in factor deficiencies. From the data shown in

Fig. 2 we calculated the prothrombin time ratios for Thromboplastin FS and MCT (ratio = dilution normal pool in sec./normal pool in sec.). The ratios of both thromboplastins were virtually equal which means that their sensitivities to factor deficiency seem to be equal.

The behaviour of anticoagulated patients also should be comparable. The therapeutic range for anticoagulated patients monitored by MCT has been established as ratio 2-4, which corresponds to 12.5% - 30% activity.

Loeliger (1) calculated the therapeutic range for Thromboplastin FS by comparison with Thrombotest and found 17% - 28% activity or 2.1 - 3.1 ratio.

Duckert has found a range of 14% - 27% for Thromboplastin FS, calculated by comparison with Human Brain Thromboplastin Basel (1).

Until now we recommended for Thromboplastin FS a therapeutic range of 14% - 27% or 2.2 - 3.7 ratio. Regarding only factor deficiency one would expect the same therapeutic range for MCT and FS.

3.2.2. <u>Study with 230 long-term anticoagulated patients</u>. The prothrombin time in the plasma of 230 anticoagulated patients was measured by MCT and FS.

In fig. 3 we plotted the PT's of the two reagents (y = FS in seconds; x = MCT in seconds). The figure demonstrates, that MCT-values differ from FS-values. The more intensely the patient is anticoagulated the more different are the compared values from x = y (curve III). Curve I shows the linear regression line (y = 6.23 + 0.68 x, r^2 = 0.98). Because we thought that the power function $y = a\ x^b$ would give us a better regression line we calculated a line of $y = 2.01\ x^{0.76}$, r^2 = 0.97. Both the calculations and visual inspection of the data points show that anticoagulated patients differ from the expected behaviour MCT = FS (x = y).

3.2.3. <u>Statistical analysis of the patient group</u>. We classified the patients in 5 groups according to PT's determined with MCT. Beside the PT's in seconds for MCT and FS the ratios (pa-

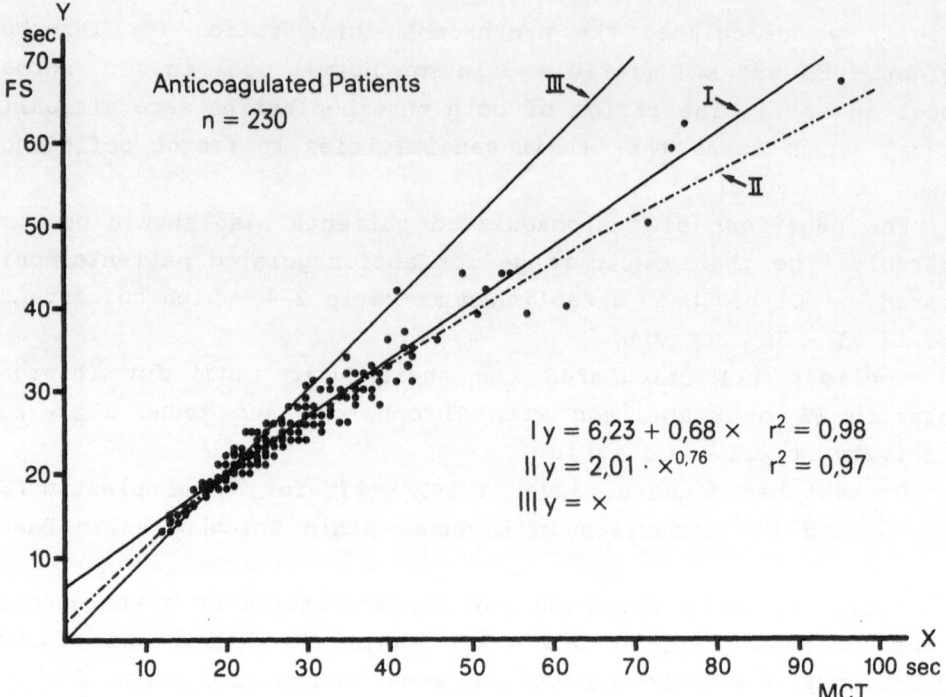

FIGURE 3: Comparison of prothrombin times for Thromboplastin FS (y-axis) with prothrombin times for Manchester Comparative Thromboplastin (x-axis), measured in 230 patients treated with oral anticoagulants.

tient plasma in sec./normal pool in sec.) are presented (normal pool: MCT = 12.5 seconds; FS = 13.5 seconds).

The ranges of the five patient groups are:
    a.   10 - 20 seconds   MCT = 0.8 - 1.6 ratio
    b.   20 - 25 seconds   MCT = 1.6 - 2.0 ratio
    c.   25 - 30 seconds   MCT = 2.0 - 2.4 ratio
    d.   30 - 40 seconds   MCT = 2.4 - 3.2 ratio
    e.   > 40 seconds   MCT   > 3.2 ratio

The values measured with Thromboplastin FS are compared with the MCT-values. For each patient group, we calculated the regression line by the method of Passing and Bablok (2) and also the ratio of the mean values ($\bar{x}$) of MCT to Thromboplastin FS.

Table 2

Patient group	n	PT in seconds		PT ratio = $\dfrac{\text{patient plasma in sec.}}{\text{normal pool in sec.}}$	
		Regression line	$\dfrac{\text{MCT sec } \bar{x}}{\text{FS sec } x}$	Regression line	$\dfrac{\text{MCT ratio } \bar{x}}{\text{FS ratio } x}$
a.	47	y = 2.5+0.875x	0.98	y = 0.09+0.911x	1.01
b.	65	y = -1.0+1.0x	1.04	y = -0.15+1.0x	1.08
c.	52	y = -2.0+1.0x	1.09	y = -0.28+1.0x	1.13
d.	46	y = 0.167+0.833x	1.18	y = 0.145+0.75x	1.22
e.	19	y = 4.21+0.72x	1.28	y = 0.32+0.69x	1.33

n = number of patients

The statistical analysis shows the changes of PT's with MCT and FS in relation to increasing anticoagulation intensity very well. Whereas MCT and FS show similar relationships when only factor deficiency is regarded (fig. 2), the anticoagulated patient data show a difference.

In conclusion we see that the difference in prothrombin times and their ratios between MCT and FS increases from 1% for MCT-ratio < 1.6 (> 40% activity) up to 33% for MCT-ratio > 3.2 (< 15.7% activity). The deviation from linearity (x = y) was calculated as significant at a low anticoagulation level under ratio 2.0 by the Cusum test (cumulated sum) (2).

In a histogram (fig. 4) we visualize the differences in PT's of the 230 anticoagulated patients measured by MCT (fig. 4A) and Thromboplastin FS (fig. 4B).

4. DISCUSSION

Because the factor sensitivity of MCT and FS is similar (FS is even more sensitive than MCT), it seems quite clear to us that, when using MCT for prothrombin time determination in anticoagulated patients, we measure other influences in addition to the anticoagulation-dependent decrease of coagulation factors. We

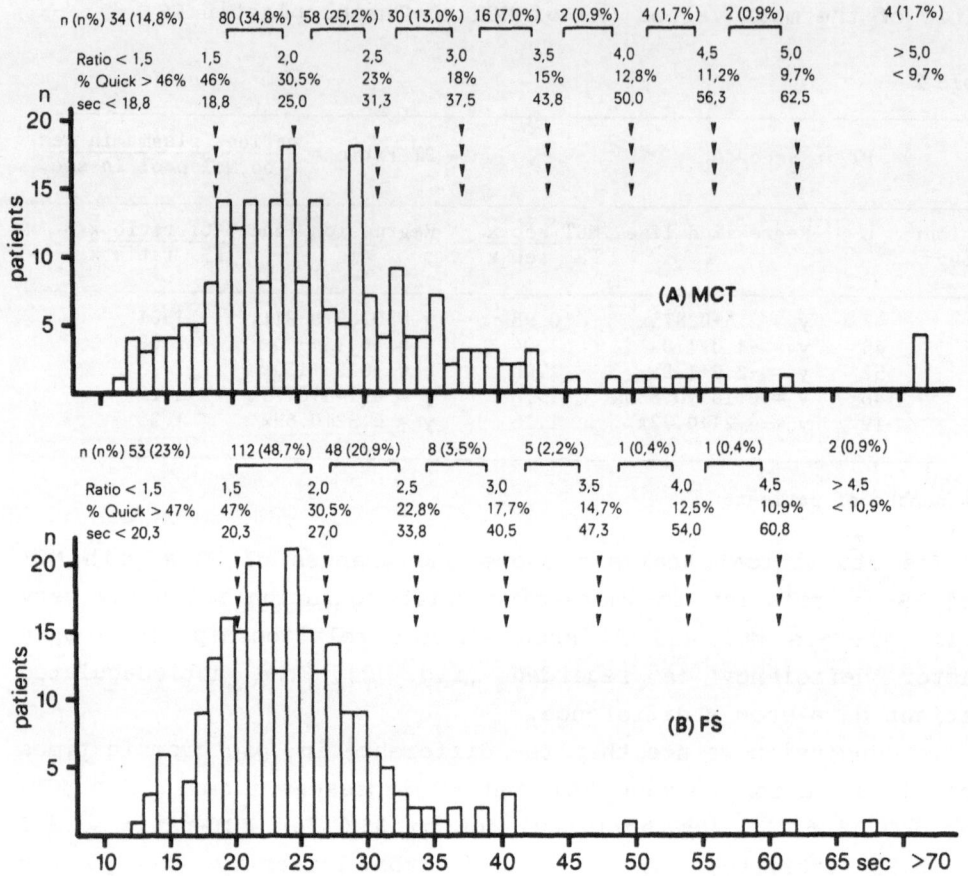

FIGURE 4: Histogram of prothrombin times of 230 patients treated with oral anticoagulants. A: Manchester Comparative Thromboplastin. B: Thromboplastin FS.

think our study shows that the differences between these reagents are not due to factor VII- or factor X-sensitivity problems but to Proteins Induced by Vitamin K Antagonists (PIVKAs).

5. SUMMARY

We compared Dade Thromboplastin FS, a rabbit brain thromboplastin highly sensitive to coagulation factor deficiencies, with two human brain preparations. It was shown that FS is as factor sensitive as Human Brain Thromboplastin Basel. Furthermore, a linear relationship between prothrombin time ratios with FS and Human Brain Thromboplastin Basel was found (calibration constant of FS vs. Human Brain Thromboplastin Basel was assessed at 0.986).

The human brain preparation Manchester Comparative Thromboplastin (MCT) is less factor sensitive than FS, the reaction to normals and to dilutions of normal plasma was quite similar but anticoagulated patients showed differences. The more anticoagulant a patient received the longer the PT became when measured with MCT in comparison to FS. We think that MCT measured not only the deficiency of carboxylated coagulation factors, but also the sub- or non-carboxylated factors (PIVKA). Therefore it is not possible to use one conversion factor over the whole range for normals, patients with factor deficiencies and anticoagulated patients. For patients treated with vitamin K-antagonists we need several conversion factors because the differences between the reagents increase with the anticoagulation intensity. The result of this study will be published in more detailed form (4).

REFERENCES

1. Duckert F, Marbet GA, Beeser H, Gouault-Heilmann M, Loeliger EA. Suitability of Thromboplastin FS for the control of oral anticoagulation. VIIth International Congress on Thrombosis and Hemostasis, London 1979.

2. Passing H, Bablok W. Application of Linear Regression Procedures in Method Comparison Studies. Part 1: Deviation of a new statistical procedure. J Clin Chem Biochem 1983;21:709-720

3a. Spaethe R, Lampart A, Naumann M, Strauss J, Widmer S. Ein neues Kalibrierplasma "CoagCal^R" zur Erstellung von Eichkurven bei gerinnungsphysiologischen Untersuchungen. In: Haemostase, Thrombophilie und Arteriosklerose (Eds: Van de Loo J, Asbeck F). Schattauer Verlag 1982; 683-689.

3b. Spaethe R, Lampart A, Naumann M, Strauss J, Widmer S. A new Calibration Plasma "CoagCal^R" for the Supply of Calibration Curves in Coagulation Assays. Biologic Prospective, 5. Colloque International de Pont-A-Mousson, 1982; 345-348.

4. Spaethe R, Greber S, Lampart A, Comparison of a factor sensitive rabbit brain thromboplastin with human brain thrombo-

206

plastins. A study of 230 patients under oral anticoagulant treatment. Submitted for publication.

COMMENT ON DR. SPAETHE'S CONTRIBUTION

A.M.H.P. VAN DEN BESSELAAR

Dr. Spaethe provides very interesting data of two calibration exercises: Thromboplastin FS vs. Human Brain Thromboplastin Basel and Thromboplastin FS vs. Manchester Comparative Reagent. The data of the first study show a good fit to a linear (non-logarithmic) relationship between prothrombin time ratios. In fact, the ratios with both thromboplastins were virtually identical. In the second study a quite different situation is met: a linear (non-logarithmic) model does not describe the relationship adequately. A linear relationship is only suitable for small intervals of anticoagulation intensity and different linear regression lines have been calculated for each interval. This leads to different conversion factors for each interval of anticoagulation intensity.

In the new calibration model proposed by BCR and WHO a linear relationship is assumed between the logarithms of prothrombin times. In fact, this is equivalent to the power function $y = a\, x^b$ used by Dr. Spaethe. The power b has the same function as the ISI in the BCR/WHO model. In tabel 1 a comparison is made between the set of 5 different linear (non-logarithmic) regression lines calculated by Dr. Spaethe and a single power function. It is shown that both methods for conversion of ratios give very similar results. In conclusion, it is possible to convert ratios with a single power function. This implies that Thromboplastin FS fits into the BCR/WHO calibration system, because Manchester Comparative Reagent also fits to this system (chapter 9).

It is clear that the data of the first study (Thromboplastin FS vs. Human Brain Thromboplastin Basel) also fit a single power function (power = 1.0). It is interesting that both liver patients and patients under oral anticoagulants fit to the same relationship. It should be noted, however, that the BCR/WHO system has been developed for oral anticoagulant control only.

T A B L E 1

Comparison of linear conversion of ratios with
exponential conversion

Patient group	linear regression of ratios			power function	
	MCT-ratio (R_{MCT})	FS-ratio (R_{FS})	$\dfrac{R_{MCT}}{R_{FS}}$	$R_{FS} = (R_{MCT})^{0.82}$	$\dfrac{R_{MCT}}{R_{FS}}$
a	1.2	1.18	1.01	1.16	1.03
b	1.8	1.65	1.09	1.62	1.11
c	2.2	1.92	1.15	1.91	1.15
d	2.8	2.25	1.25	2.33	1.20
e	5.0	3.77	1.33	3.74	1.34

Chapter 12: PROFICIENCY TESTING AND STANDARDIZATION OF PRO-
THROMBIN TIME: POTENTIAL USE OF THROMBOPLASTIN
CALIBRATION IN THE UNITED STATES

D.A. TRIPLETT, B.L. EVATT and A.M.H.P. VAN DEN BESSELAAR

1. INTRODUCTION

In the past, standardization efforts aimed at the prothrombin time were mainly concerned with establishing a reference thromboplastin against which any other thromboplastin could be calibrated. Such calibration was based upon the empiric model developed by Biggs and Denson (1). Reproducible calibration could be achieved by testing many plasma samples from patients treated with oral anticoagulants. More recently, Loeliger's laboratory has shown that under certain conditions, lyophilized pooled plasmas could replace fresh patient plasmas for use in calibration of thromboplastins (2).

The underlying premise of such a calibration scheme identified thromboplastins as the primary cause of deviation of a prothrombin time measured in one test system (i.e. reagent/instrument) as compared to a prothrombin time measured in another. This is certainly true when dealing with prothrombin time test systems that use different classes of thromboplastins, for instance, thromboplastins of rabbit tissue origin commonly used in the United States vs. those prepared from human tissue like British Comparative Thromboplastin. However, in inter-laboratory surveys where prothrombin time results are grouped according to tissue origin of thromboplastin, the influence of the thromboplastin is reduced. Another important variable which has not been fully appreciated is the type of laboratory instrumentation used in determining the prothrombin time. In early studies done as a result of collaboration between the College of American Pathologists and the Centers for Disease Control, it was found that the type of instrument used in performing the prothrombin time has almost as much an effect as the type of thromboplastin (3). In addition, both of these variables added together accounted for approximately half of the inter-laboratory variation. The mathematical relationships derived from the above study suggested further useful applications; therefore, some of the details of that initial study will be presented.

2. ADDITIVE MODEL OF PROTHROMBIN TIME

For the study, a data base generally being accumulated by the College of American Pathologists (CAP) Proficiency Testing Program was examined. This examination provided data from 2,735 laboratories taking part in the CAP Survey Program in 1977. Plasma was collected from plasmaphoresis donors and specimens which were designated to have prolonged prothrombin times were artificially depleted of vitamin K-dependent coagulation factors by aluminum hydroxide adsorption. Three different pools were established representing normal, intermediately prolonged and very prolonged prothrombin times. These samples were inserted in the routine survey mailing and sent to the participating laboratories. Each laboratory was instructed to use its routine instrument and thromboplastin in measuring prothrombin times on the three plasma samples. Participants in the survey used 12 different standard instruments and 12 different standard thromboplastins resulting in a total of 144 possible system combinations. Not all of these systems were actually used by the laboratories in the survey and for the purposes of data analysis, 8 thromboplastins and 7 instruments for a total of 56 different combinations of thromboplastins and instruments formed the data base which could be analyzed according to two-way analysis of variance by the program ANOVA in Statistical Package for the Social Sciences (option, classical experimental approach) (4). Using a general linear model approach to a non-orthogonal analysis of variance, two-way interaction was tested first for statistical significance before testing for significance of the main effects. Clearly, interaction between the instruments and the thromboplastins could be ignored for practical purposes and a simple additive model for plasma samples was used. This model appeared to be a very effective predictor of the instrument and thromboplastin effect for all the instrument and thromboplastin combinations studied (see appendix for statistical methods). From these data the effects of each instrument and thromboplastin on the prothrombin time were calculated (Figures 1 and 2).

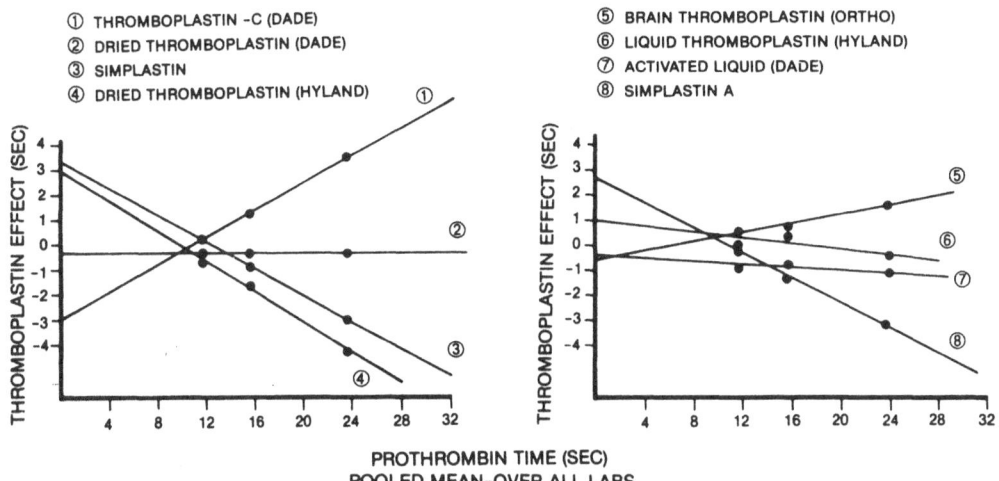

PROTHROMBIN TIME (SEC)
POOLED MEAN-OVER ALL LABS

FIGURE 1. Estimated effects for thromboplastins for three plasma samples. For each thromboplastin, the estimated effects of thromboplastin on the prothrombin time (obtained from the two-way analysis of variance performed on each sample) were plotted against the mean prothrombin time for each sample. The three points for each thromboplastin fall on or very near a straight line. (Reproduced with permission from Clin Lab Haematol 1981; 3: 331-342.)

It is important to emphasize that the estimates of each effect are in reference to the overall mean prothrombin time for all laboratories which measured the plasma samples. With a different set of thromboplastins and instruments than those used in this study, the estimates of the effect of any thromboplastin or instrument may change dramatically. Furthermore, it is important to stress that the overall prothrombin time is an unweighted mean of these laboratories, thus, the mean prothrombin time is influenced more by the fibrometer[®] than by the Clotek since about 1475 laboratories used the fibrometer[®] in this early study and only 75 laboratories used the Clotek.

212

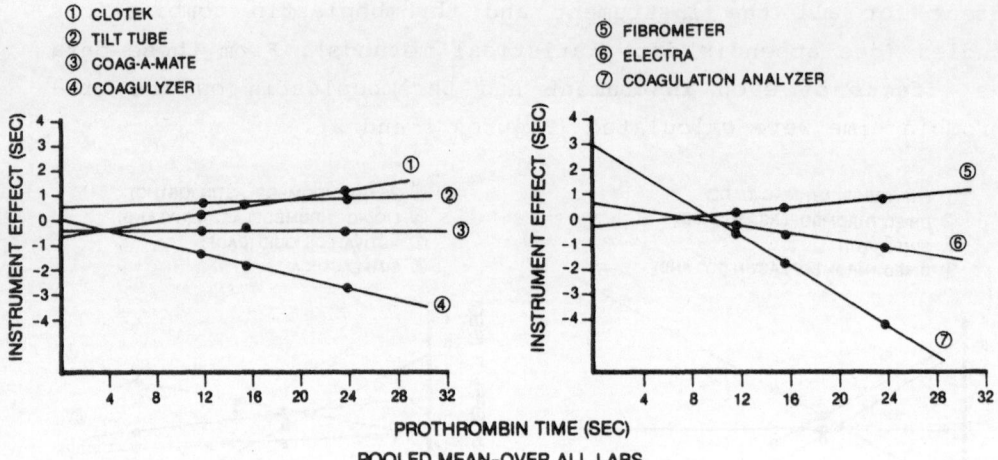

FIGURE 2. Estimated effects for instruments for three plasma samples. For each instrument, the estimated effects of instrument on the prothrombin time (obtained from the two-way analysis of variance performed on each sample) were plotted against the mean prothrombin time for each sample. The three points for each instrument fall on or very near a straight line. (Reproduced with permission from Clin Lab Haematol 1981; 3: 331-342.)

3. PROTHROMBIN TIME CORRECTION BY ADDITIVE MODEL

The results of this study suggested that a universal scale for the prothrombin time could be developed by application of these data. The corrections for instruments and thromboplastins were applied to three sets of proficiency testing data obtained in 1976, 1977, and 1978. The plotted means for any specific instrument thromboplastin combination obtained from proficiency testing surveys performed in these years showed a widely dispersed distribution (Figure 3). If on the other hand, these prothrombin times were corrected to remove the effect of each instrument and thromboplastin used in the various combinations, there was a significant decrease in variance. In fact, the mean of each instrument thromboplastin combination was within one and one-half seconds of the overall mean, a perfectly acceptable range for monitoring of anticoagulant therapy.

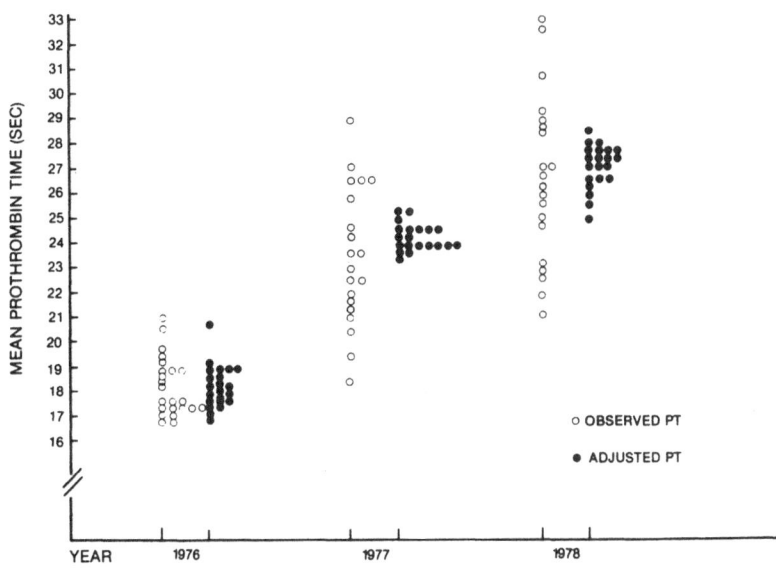

FIGURE 3. Mean observed and adjusted prothrombin time for laboratories using a given instrument/thromboplastin combination for
three proficiency testing surveys. Prothrombin times were obtained on three additional data sets obtained from CAP surveys on
the prothtombin time performed in 1976, 1977, and 1978. The
plotted means of instrument/thromboplastin combinations of the
observed data are shown in open circles and show a widely dispersed distribution. The prothrombin times from each of the
surveys were then adjusted/corrected using equation (5) (see
appendix: statistical methods) to reduce the effect of instrument
and thromboplastin and plotted using black circles. The use of
the adjustment/correction produced a significant decrease in
variance of the means of the instrument/thromboplastin combinations. (Reproduced with permission from Clin Lab Haematol 1981;
3: 331-342.)

4. REPRODUCIBILITY AND EFFECT OF PLASMA TYPE

From this early study, however, two important questions remain
to be answered. First, were the relationships for thromboplastins
and instruments reproducible from survey to survey and secondly,
were the relationships obtained by using artificially depleted
plasma the same as relationships measured from plasma derived
from patients treated with oral anticoagulants. Consequently, a
second study was undertaken by Van den Besselaar et al. to answer
these questions (5). For this study, normal plasma was obtained

by plasmaphoresis and the abnormal plasmas were manufactured by adsorption of the clotting factors with aluminum hydroxide. Also, three lyophilized patient plasmas (patients receiving oral anticoagulants) were obtained from Dr. E.A. Loeliger. The data analyzed in this study were accumulated from the proficiency testing programs conducted by the Centers for Disease Control over the period 1978-1981. In addition, data from one survey organized by the College of American Pathologists were analyzed (1978). The survey data were subjected to the same non-orthogonal two-way analysis of variance as described for the initial' study. For each plasma sample, the thromboplastin and instrument effects were estimated and computed into the linear additive model. As with the earlier study, the primary effects of thromboplastin and instrument were the main effects upon the prothrombin time and there was little evidence of interaction between the two, thus allowing the interaction to be ignored. The results of this study indicated that the relationship between grand mean prothrombin time and the effect of each instrument after adjustment for any thromboplastin effect and similar data for thromboplastin effect after adjustment for any instrument effect were similar in all surveys. Several interesting observations were noted, however. For instance, in the normal and artificially depleted plasmas prepared by the CDC there was generally good correlation between grand mean and estimated effects and isolated divergent results were rare. It appeared that the position of such aberrant esti- mated effects in the plot was rather independent of the sample of laboratories providing the data from which the effect was esti- mated. This suggested that the aberration was most probably due to differing composition or preparation of the plasmas used in the given survey.

In some instances, the variability of estimated effects appeared to be much larger for certain types of thromboplastins. In these instances, it was probably due to a lower number of laboratories using a particular thromboplastin. On the other hand, there was good correlation between the grand mean and estimated effects of optical instrumentation other than those explicitly identified on the returned survey forms. This suggested that the optical density instrumentation group, although poorly defined was essentially homogeneous.

In comparing the CAP and CDC sample results, the data points of the artificially depleted CAP samples diverged significantly from those of the artificially depleted CDC samples. The most obvious deviation was observed for Simplastin Automated[®] with the difference in estimated effect amounting to about 5 seconds at a grand mean value of 24 seconds.

In comparing the data obtained on plasmas from patients who were adequately anticoagulated, there was a difference from the artificially depleted plasma. This difference was seen with several thromboplastins; the most obvious being noted for Simplastin[®].

The conclusions from this study were similar to those of the earlier study of Evatt et al. (3). Although in most cases there was a significant interaction between instrument and thromboplas-

Table 1   Mean and coefficient of variation of reported prothrombin times and corrected prothrombin times of artificially depleted plasma for an unweighted mean over all labs (section A) and an equally weighted mean of 33 instrument/thromboplastin combinations (section B). Correction of individual prothrombin times was performed by equation (5) (see appendix). The parameters in this equation were derived from 8 normal and 10 artificially depleted plasma samples used in 8 surveys.

	n	reported prothrombin time mean (sec)	CV (%)	corrected prothrombin time mean (sec)	CV (%)
section A	473	20.1	10.4	20.1	8.6
section B	33	20.1	8.0	20.2	3.3

tin, it was minor and the data could be described by a linear additive mathematical model. Furthermore, the systematic differences in prothrombin time between thromboplastins and instruments were reduced by correcting the prothrombin times by means of this model (Table 1). It is also clear that the composition and origin of plasma may determine the relationship between the grand mean and estimated effect. When the observed prothrombin times of a patient (coumadinized) sample are corrected by parameters derived from adsorbed plasma, the reduction in variance is much less in comparison with a correction by parameters derived from coumadinized patient plasma (Table 2).

Table 2   Mean and coefficient of variation of reported prothrombin times and corrected prothrombin times of pooled patient plasma (patients treated with oral anticoagulants) for an equally weighted mean of 36 instrument/thromboplastin combinations. Individual prothrombin times were corrected by equation 5 (see appendix). Correction was performed with two sets of parameters: the first set was derived from data of normal and artificially depleted plasma samples; the second set was obtained from data of a normal and two pooled patient plasma samples.

	mean (sec)	CV (%)
reported prothrombin time	20.8	10.6
corrected prothrombin time (artificial plasma parameters)	21.2	9.6
corrected prothrombin time (patient plasma parameters)	21.2	3.7

5. STANDARDIZATION BY THE ADDITIVE MODEL AND ITS LINK WITH THE WHO SYSTEM

The aim of standardization is to convert prothrombin times of individual patients treated with oral anticoagulants to a common scale. The linear additive model may be used for standardization. It has the advantage that both thromboplastin and instrument effects are accounted for. Conversion of prothrombin times to the level of a grand mean should not be recommended since the grand mean is still dependent upon the distribution of instruments and thromboplastins. This influence can be eliminated if the prothrombin time is converted to the time which would be obtained with that of a particular instrument and thromboplastin combination. This implies, however, that a particular instrument thromboplastin combination would be considered as a reference method; a designation which may lead to problems in selecting a standard.

Since this study demonstrated that patient plasmas have different properties when compared with artificially depleted plasmas, standardization should be based upon patient plasma. Several investigators have suggested that the bias due to different instruments could be eliminated more or less by the use of ratios of abnormal prothrombin to normal prothrombin times (6). The use of such ratios has two drawbacks. First, the experimental error of the normal values is added to that of the abnormal value. In addition, a second bias may be produced because there are many normal controls and no generally accepted standards for normal plasma.

The model described would be complementary to standardization based on ratios proposed by the WHO (7). In fact, only one additional table of conversion would be required to transform standardized prothrombin times into International Normalized Ratios (INR) as the link between both systems. Alternatively, an additional set of parameters could be calculated for a direct transformation of prothrombin times determined with any thromboplastin instrument combination into International Normalized Ratios.

REFERENCES

1. Biggs R, Denson KWE. Standardization of the one stage prothrombin time for the control of anticoagulant therapy. Br Med J 1967; 1: 84.
2. Loeliger EA, Van Halem-Visser LP. A simplified thromboplastin calibration procedure for standardization of anticoagulant control. Thromb Diath Haemorrh 1975; 33: 172.
3. Evatt BL, Brogan D, Triplett DA, Waters G. Effect of thromboplastin and instrumentation on the prothrombin time test. Clin Lab Haematol 1981; 3: 331.
4. Kim JO, Kohout FJ. Analysis of variance and covariance: Subprograms ANOVA and one-way. In: Nie NH, Hull CH, Jenkins JF, Stein-Brenner K and Bent DH (Eds.): Statistical Package for the Social Sciences. McGraw-Hill, New York 1975, 2nd ed.: p. 398.
5. Van den Besselaar AMHP, Evatt BL, Brogan DR, Triplett DA. Proficiency testing and standardization of prothrombin time: Effect of thromboplastin, instrumentation and plasma. Submitted for publication.
6. Koepke JA, Gilmer PR, Triplett DA, O'Sullivan MB. The prediction of prothrombin time system performance using secondary standards. Am J Clin Pathol 1977; 68: 191.

218

7. World Health Organization Expert Committee on Biological Standardization. Thirty-third Report. Technical Report Series 687. WHO, Geneva 1983: pp. 81-105.

APPENDIX

Statistical methods

The statistical model ·and analysis are the same as used in Evatt et al. (3), a brief summary of which is given here. The linear additive model for prothrombin time for a given plasma sample m in a given survey is described as

$$Y_{ijkm} = m_m + \alpha_{im} + \beta_{jm} + \varepsilon_{ijkm} \qquad \text{(equation 1)}$$

where

Y_{ijkm} = reported prothrombin time for plasma sample m from laboratory k using instrument i and thromboplastin j

μ_m = mean prothrombin time for plasma sample m over all laboratories

α_{im} = instrument effect for plasma m

β_{jm} = thromboplastin effect for plasma m

ε_{ijkm} = random error term.

In any particular survey there are two or more plasma samples, (i.e. $m \geq 2$), and n_{ijm} labs who respond to plasma m by using thromboplastin j and instrument i.

Evatt et al. (3) found that the linear model in equation (1) fits well, not requiring any interaction terms, for the three plasma levels in their one survey (multiple R^2 ranged from 42% to 58%).

When the actual instrument and thromboplastin effects α_{im} and β_{jm} were estimated by Evatt et al. (3), they found a strong linear relationship between the magnitude of a given effect (e.g. $\hat{\alpha}_{im}$) and the mean prothrombin time for that plasma sample (i.e. $\hat{\mu}_m$). Thus, each effect was modeled as a linear function of μ_m as

$$\alpha_{im} = \gamma_i \mu_m + \kappa_i \qquad \text{(equation 2)}$$

$$\beta_{jm} = \delta_j \mu_m + \xi_j \qquad \text{(equation 3)}$$

where μ_m is the mean prothrombin time. Substituting equations (2) and (3) into (1) yields

$$y_{ijkm} = \mu_m(1 + \gamma_i + \delta_j) + (\kappa_i + \xi_j) + \varepsilon_{ijkm} \qquad \text{(equation 4)}$$

The "corrected" prothrombin time corresponds to the parameter μ_m in equation (4) and is estimated by y'_{ijkm}, where

$$y'_{ijkm} = \frac{y_{ijkm} - (\hat{\kappa}_i + \hat{\xi}_j)}{(1 + \hat{\gamma}_i + \hat{\delta}_j)} \qquad \text{(equation 5)}$$

where $\hat{\kappa}_i$, $\hat{\xi}_j$, $\hat{\gamma}_i$ and $\hat{\delta}_j$ are the estimated slopes and intercepts from equations (2) and (3). (Note that the error term ε_{ijkm} has been ignored.)

From all individually corrected prothrombin times y'_{ijkm} in a survey a grand mean for a given plasma sample m can be calculated as $\bar{y}'_m$ where

$$\bar{y}'_m = \frac{1}{n} \sum_{k=1}^{n} y'_{ijkm} \qquad \text{(equation 6)}$$

where n is the number of laboratories in the survey who responded to plasma m. The variation (standard deviation) in the y'_{ijkm}, for given m, is calculated as

$$s'_m = \left[\sum_{k=1}^{n} (y'_{ijkm} - \bar{y}'_m)^2 / (n - 1) \right]^{\frac{1}{2}} \qquad \text{(equation 7)}$$

Reported prothrombin times y_{ijkm} can also be transformed or corrected to prothrombin times that whould have been obtained with instrument c and thromboplastin t. Such transformation is obtained by eliminating μ_m from the two appropriate equations (4) and ignoring terms ε_{ijkm} and ε_{ctkm}

$$y^*_{ctkm} = \{y_{ijkm} - (\hat{\kappa}_i + \hat{\xi}_j)\}\frac{(1+\hat{\gamma}_c+\hat{\delta}_t)}{(1+\hat{\gamma}_i+\hat{\delta}_j)} + (\hat{\kappa}_c + \hat{\xi}_t) \qquad \text{(equation 8)}$$

When all transformed prothrombin times as in equation (8) are averaged over all reporting labs, the mean $\bar{y}^*_{ctm}$ is calculated as

$$\bar{y}^\star_{ctm} = \frac{1}{n} \sum_{k=1}^{n} y^\star_{ctkm} \qquad\qquad \text{(equation 9)}$$

where n is the number of laboratories in the survey who responded to plasma m.

Survey data were subjected to a non-orthogonal two-way analysis of variance as described by Evatt et al (3). For this purpose the program ANOVA in SPSS (Statistical Package for Social Sciences) was used with the option called the "Classical experimental approach" (4).

Chapter 13: THE RELATIONSHIP BETWEEN THE INTERNATIONAL NORMAL-
IZED RATIO AND THE COUMARIN-INDUCED COAGULATION
DEFECT

R.M. BERTINA

1. INTRODUCTION

For the laboratory monitoring of patients treated with oral
anticoagulants it is of great importance that a common scale or
international unit exists in which a prothrombin time - determined with any of the many different thromboplastin preparations - can be expressed. Recently such a common scale has become
available by the introduction of the International Normalized
Ratio (INR) as the international unit for the coumarin-induced
coagulation defect (1). The concept of INR has been developed
within the framework of prothrombin time standardisation. However, its application will not be limited to the standardisation
of the prothrombin time. In fact, the INR will be of great importance for the standardisation of all laboratory assays and determinations that can be used for the monitoring of oral anticoagulant therapy.

There are several reasons why we are interested in the relation between the INR and the actual coagulation defect induced by
the anti-vitamin K drugs:
a) it may lead to a definition/description of INR in terms of
biochemical parameters;
b) it will allow a better definition of pooled patient plasmas,
that are intended to be used in thromboplastin calibration;
c) it will be possible to provide reliable therapeutic ranges for
the laboratory monitoring of oral anticoagulant treatment with
single factor assays.

224

2. ACTION OF VITAMIN K ANTAGONISTS

Figure 1 schematically shows how anti-vitamin K drugs interfere with the biosynthesis of vitamin K-dependent coagulation
factors in the liver. During oral anticoagulation, the coumarin
inhibits the catalytic activity of the carboxylases involved in
the final completion of the synthesis of some of the coagulation
factors. A reduction in carboxylase activity leads to incomplete
carboxylation of these factors. Consequently, the concentration
of fully carboxylated factors (C) will decrease, while the concentrations of subcarboxylated (B) and non-carboxylated (A) factors -- also referred to as PIVKAs (2) -- will increase. The
present hypothesis is that only fully carboxylated factors have
procoagulant activity and that some of the partially carboxylated
or non-carboxylated factors may behave as competitive substrates
or inhibitors in the reactions involved in thrombin generation.

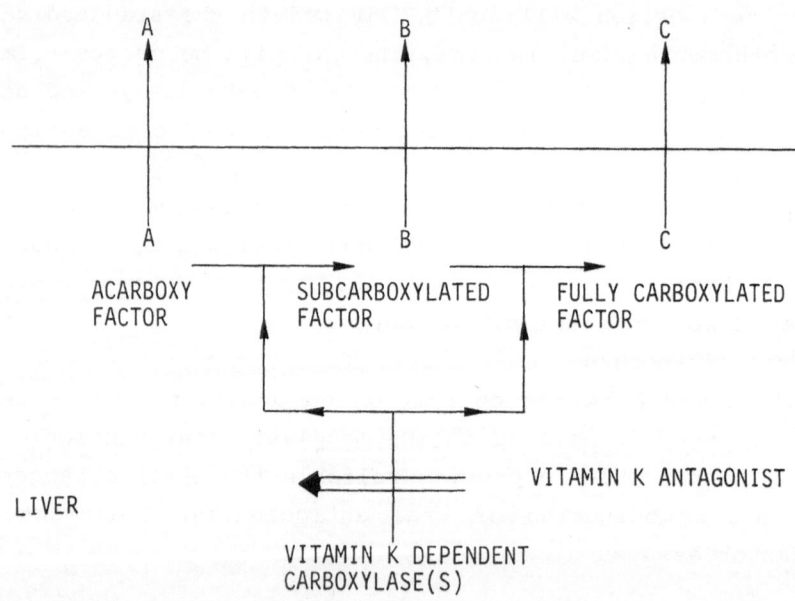

FIGURE 1. Inhibition of coagulation factor synthesis by vitamin K
antagonist.

3. MONITORING OF THE INTENSITY OF ORAL ANTICOAGULANT THERAPY

It is evident that changes in the steady state plasma concentrations of the A, B and C forms of the various vitamin K-dependent factors (see Fig. 1) will depend on the concentration of the vitamin K antagonist and thus on the intensity of the anticoagulant treatment. In clinical practice, the intensity of the treatment is monitored in the laboratory by the result of a prothrombin time determination. However, the sensitivity of the individual thromboplastins to the coumarin-induced coagulation defect may differ largely, for instance due to differences in sensitivity to:

a) factor VII and/or activated factor VII (3,4);
b) PIVKA forms (5);
c) factor IX;
d) protein C.

The sensitivity of the prothrombin time to factor IX has been demonstrated by Ørstavik and Laake (6) in case of the ox-brain thromboplastin time. Addition of anti-factor IX serum to plasma resulted in a 10% decrease in prothrombin time. This has been explained as the result of a competition between factor IX and factor X for binding to the factor VII thromboplastin complex (7). Differences in sensitivity to protein C levels might be of importance, now that significant amounts of thrombomodulin have been demonstrated in some thromboplastin preparations (Bertina and Van Wijngaarden, unpublished observations); thrombomodulin binds thrombin effectively and thus greatly accelerates the activation of protein C (8); activated protein C is a potent inhibitor of the prothrombin time by its inactivation of activated factor V (9). Moreover, the thrombomodulin-thrombin complex cannot clot fibrinogen (10).

At present it is possible to convert the prothrombin time determined with one thromboplastin into a normalized ratio (INR) that in turn can be converted into the prothrombin time that would have been obtained with any other thromboplastin. This makes the INR the ideal parameter for the quantitation of the intensity of oral anticoagulant treatment.

4. VITAMIN K-DEPENDENT COAGULATION FACTORS

Seven plasma proteins are known to contain the characteristic vitamin K dependent structure (γ-carboxy glutamic acid residues) at the aminoterminal part of the molecule or its light chain: factors II, VII, IX and X, protein C (11), protein S (12) and protein Z (13). Protein S seems to be involved in blood coagulation as a cofactor of activated protein C (14). The function of protein Z is still not known.

Table 1: Specificity of assays of vitamin K-dependent factors

assay	fully carboxylated	partially carboxylated	non-carboxylated
coagulation	+	?	-/inhibitor
spectrophotometric	+	+/?	-/?
RIA	+	+/-	+/-
Laurell	+	+/-	+/-
INA	+	+	+
ELISA	+	+/-	+/-

Several types of assay are available for the quantitative estimation of the concentration of a vitamin K-dependent factor in plasma. Table 1 summarizes to which degree these different assays are supposed to be specific for the fully carboxylated, partially carboxylated and non-carboxylated forms of the proteins. Especially in case of the immunologic assays, it is insufficiently known how partially carboxylated and non-carboxylated forms behave. But also for some of the spectrophotometric assays (factor X, protein C) it is still questionable to what degree partially carboxylated forms are co-assayed.

In our laboratory we use the following assays for the vitamin K-dependent coagulation factors: factor VII and factor IX activity: one stage coagulation assays (15,16); factor II, factor X and protein C activity: spectrophotometric assays (17,18,19); factor II, factor IX, factor X and protein C antigen: electro-immunoassay (20,21); factor VII antigen: inhibitor neutralisation assay (20).

5. PATIENT MATERIALS

To study the relationship between the INR and the coumarin-induced coagulation defect, we used:
a) the plasmas of 150 stably anticoagulated patients, and
b) pools of plasmas of stably anticoagulated patients.
In all cases the INR was calculated from the prothrombin time determined within 2 hours after venepuncture.

The study has been limited to plasmas of patients who were stably anticoagulated because the INR has been defined on the basis of prothrombin times determined in plasmas of stable patients (1).

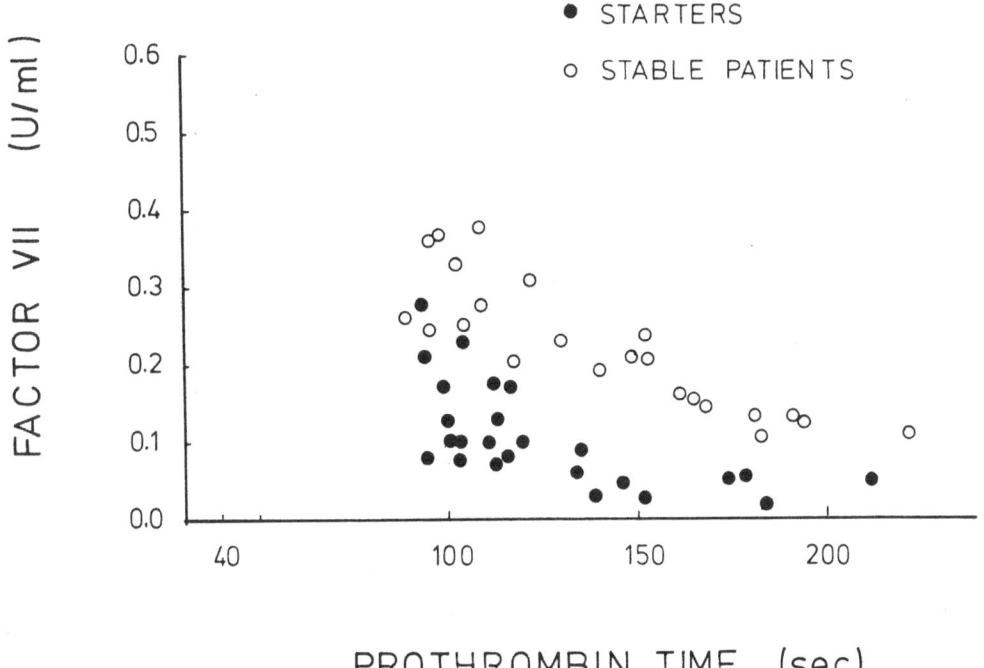

FIGURE 2. Relationship between prothrombin time (Thrombotest) and factor VII activity

We know from previous studies that the relationship between the prothrombin time and the concentration of the vitamin K-dependent factors varies largely with the degree of stability of the patient. Figure 2 for example shows the relationship between factor VII activity and prothrombin time for a group of stably anticoagulated patients and for a group of patients who have been treated for a period shorter than 10 days (Starters). It is evident that at the same prothrombin time, the starters have a much lower factor VII concentration than the stable patients.

According to our definition, a stably anticoagulated patient at the time of control has an INR within the therapeutic range, while the change in INR (when compared with that of the previous control) is less than 0.75%/day; also at the two preceding controls the INR should have been in the therapeutic range.

6. RELATIONSHIP BETWEEN INR AND COUMARIN-INDUCED COAGULATION DEFECT

6.1. Analysis of plasmas of individual patients

Table 2: Relationship between INR and Factor II (spectrophotometric assay). N = number of patients

INR	N	C(+) (U/ml)	$\frac{C(+)}{A + B + C}$
2.70	17	0.28 ± 0.04	0.52 ± 0.06
3.00	36	0.23 ± 0.04	0.45 ± 0.09
3.40	35	0.19 ± 0.04	0.38 ± 0.07
3.75	18	0.18 ± 0.05	0.37 ± 0.10
4.25	18	0.155 ± 0.03	0.32 ± 0.07
4.71	26	0.125 ± 0.03	0.29 ± 0.07

Table 2 summarizes data that have been obtained for factor II. The 150 individual plasmas were distributed over 6 different INR intervals. Within each interval, mean values were calculated for the INR and in this case for factor II, as measured spectrophotometrically (this is called C(+) in table 2). The ratio C(+)/A+B+C has been calculated from the ratio between the result of the spectrophotometric assay and the result of the immunologic assay (which is supposed to measure A+B+C, see Fig. 1). This ratio gives the fraction of the factor II molecules that has procoagulant activity, for each INR value. With increasing INR -- i.e., with increasing intensity of anticoagulation -- not only factor II activity (C+) decreases, but also the fraction of factor II molecules that have procoagulant activity.

Table 3: Relation between INR and factor II, factor X, factor VII and factor IX activity

INR	$\overline{\text{F II}}$ (U/ml)	$\overline{\text{F X}}$ (U/ml)	$\overline{\text{F VII}}$ (U/ml)	$\overline{\text{F IX}}$ (U/ml)
2.70	0.28 ±0.04	0.22 ±0.04	0.37±0.13	0.42±0.07
3.00	0.23 ±0.04	0.20 ±0.04	0.36±0.11	0.39±0.07
3.40	0.19 ±0.04	0.18 ±0.04	0.27±0.08	0.33±0.06
3.75	0.18 ±0.05	0.17 ±0.04	0.24±0.06	0.30±0.07
4.25	0.155±0.03	0.155±0.03	0.20±0.05	0.25±0.08
4.71	0.125±0.04	0.155±0.03	0.16±0.04	0.21±0.05

In Table 3, mean values for factors II, VII, IX and X activity have been compared at different INR values. At most INR values, factor VII and factor IX are significantly higher than factors II and X. All activities decrease with increasing INR. The reduction of factor X from 0.22 U/ml at INR 2.70 to 0.155 U/ml at INR 4.71 is much smaller than that observed for the other factors.

Using results as shown in Table 3, it will be possible to predict that, for instance, the ideal patient, anticoagulated at an intensity corresponding with an INR of 3.75, has FII = 0.18 U/ml, FX = 0.17 U/ml, FVII = 0.24 U/ml, and FX = 0.30 U/ml.

For practical purposes, however, it would be helpful if plasmas of such ideal patients, treated at different intensities of oral anticoagulant treatment, were readily available.

6.2.Analysis of pooled patient plasmas

We prepared - on small scale - pools of plasmas of patients that were stably anticoagulated with an INR within defined limits. These pools were analysed in the same way as the plasmas of the individual patients.

Table 4: Relation between INR and factor II in pooled patient plasmas. n = number of patients included in each pool.

| $\overline{INR}$* | Factor II activity (U/ml) | | | | |
	Pool I (n=10)	Pool II (n=10)	Pool III (n=10)	Pool IV (n=10)	Pool I-IV (n=40)
2.9	0.31	0.31	0.31	0.29	0.295
3.4	0.25	0.25	0.22	0.20	0.235
4.0	0.19	0.17	0.20	0.19	0.185
4.8	0.16	0.15	0.13	0.18	0.155

*$\overline{INR}$ was calculated from the INRs of the individual plasmas contributing to the pools

Table 4 shows the results obtained for factor II activity in 20 different pool plasmas. In general, there is not much difference in the factor II content of the pools with the same INR. However, sometimes differences are quite obvious: for instance at INR 3.4: pool I contains 0.25 U/ml FII, while pool IV contains only 0.20 U/ml FII, or at INR 4.8: Pool III contains 0.13 U/ml F II and pool IV 0.18 U/ml.

Table 5 and 6 show the variation in factor II, factor X, factor VII and factor IX activity between 4 different 10-donor pools with an INR of about 2.9 (Table 5) and between 4 different 10-donor pools with an INR of about 4.8 (Table 6). From analysis of data as shown in Tables 4-6, we will try to define the minimal number of donors that is necessary for the preparation of a plasma pool that can be considered as reflecting the plasma of an ideal patient at a well-defined intensity of treatment.

Table 5: Factor II, factor X, factor VII and factor IX activity in
pool plasmas with an INR of 2.9

pool plasma	N	INR	F II (U/ml)	F X (U/ml)	F VII (U/ml)	F IX (U/ml)
I	10	2.93	0.30	0.26	0.30	0.48
II	10	2.87	0.31	0.24	0.30	0.40
III	10	2.91	0.310	0.23	0.33	0.48
IV	10	2.91	0.290	0.24	0.29	0.45
I-IV	40	2.91	0.295	0.255	0.28	0.41

Table 6: Factor II, factor X, factor VII and factor IX activity in
pool plasmas with an INR of 4.8

pool plasma	N	INR	F II (U/ml)	F X (U/ml)	F VII (U/ml)	F IX (U/ml)
I	10	4.89	0.16	0.16	0.11	0.22
II	10	4.84	0.15	0.16	0.10	0.23
III	10	4.81	0.13	0.18	0.12	0.24
IV	10	4.61	0.18	0.18	0.11	0.25
I-IV	40	4.81	0.155	0.17	0.12	0.20

7. COMPARISON OF RESULTS OBTAINED IN PLASMAS OF INDIVIDUAL PATIENTS AND IN POOL PLASMAS

Figure 3 compares the relationship between the INR and factor IX activity as obtained in the 150 individual plasmas and in the 40-donor pools of plasmas of stably anticoagulated patients. In the case of factor IX there is a good agreement between the results of the two experimental approaches. However, for factor II and factor X the values measured in the pools are slightly higher than those in the individual plasmas (cf. Table 4-6, with Tables 2,3), while for factor VII slightly lower values were measured in the pools. The explanation for these discrepancies is not known presently and subject to further studies.

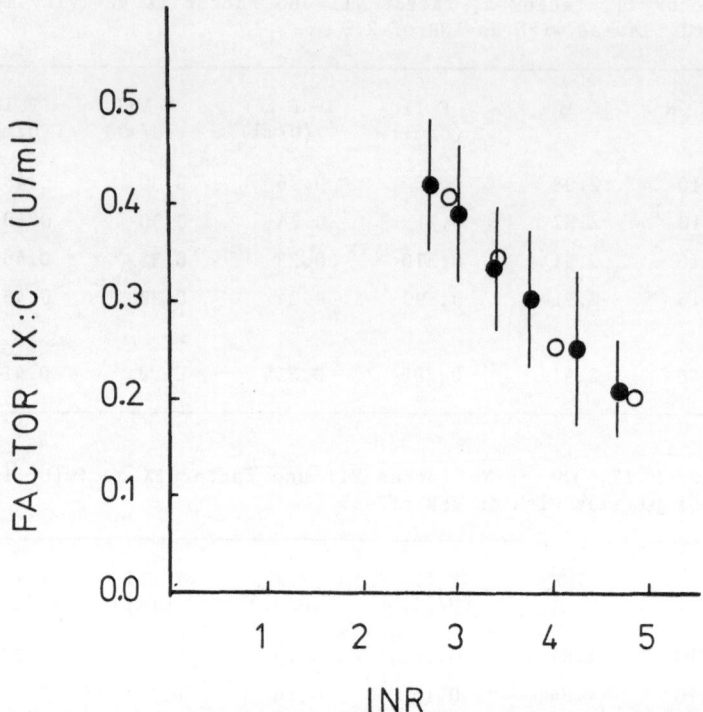

FIGURE 3: Relation between factor IX activity and INR. Individual patients are represented by closed circles with a vertical bar (mean value ± standard deviation);pooled plasmas are represented by open circles.

8. DISCUSSION

The results in Tables 2-6 demonstrate that principally it is possible to relate the INR to the coumarin-induced coagulation defect in terms of biochemical parameters. When necessary, we can define the coagulation defect in the ideal patient treated with oral anticoagulants at an intensity corresponding with a fixed INR. Table 7 gives an example for a patient with a INR of ~3.9.

However, in the future more attention needs to be paid to the specificity of the different assays used and to the discrepancy in the results obtained in individual plasmas and pooled plasmas. Moreover, it is recommended that the relation between INR and each of the coagulation factor concentrations will be established

Table 7: Coagulation defect in ideal patient treated with oral anticoagulants at an intensity corresponding with an INR of
3.9*

	activity (U/ml)	antigen (U/ml)
factor II	0.185	0.47
factor VII	0.185	0.42
factor IX	0.250	0.42
factor X	0.190	0.33
protein C	0.260	0.48

*data are based on the results obtained in the analysis of 40-donor
pools

in a multi-centre study. Once the relationship between the INR
and the coagulation defect has been established, it will be possible to produce patient-pool plasmas with a certified INR value.
The value of such plasmas will be that they can be used both in
the standardisation of laboratory assays for the monitoring of
oral anticoagulant treatment and for the definition of the therapeutic ranges to be used for each particular assay.

REFERENCES

1. Loeliger EA, Lewis SM. Progress in laboratory control of oral
   anticoagulants. Lancet 1982; 2: 318-320.
2. Hemker HC, Veltkamp JJ, Loeliger EA, Kinetic aspects of the
   interaction of blood clotting enzymes III. Demonstration of
   an inhibitor of prothrombin conversion in vitamin K deficiency. Thromb Diathes Haemorrh 1968; 19: 346-363.
3. Hemker HC, Muller AD, Gonggrijp R. The estimation of activated human blood coagulation factor VII. J Mol Med 1976; 1:
   127-134.
4. Van Deijk WA, Van Dam-Mieras MCE, Muller AD, Hemker HC. Evaluation of a coagulation assay determining the activity state
   of factor VII in plasma. Haemostasis 1983; 13: 192-197.
5. Loeliger EA, Van Halem-Visser LP. Biological properties of
   the thromboplastins and plasmas included in the ICTH/ICSH
   collaborative study on prothrombin time standardization.
   Thromb Haemostas 1979; 42: 1115-1127.
6. Ørstavik KH, Laake K. Antiserum against factor IX shortens
   the bovine thromboplastin coagulation time of human plasma.
   Thromb Res 1978; 12: 455-465.
7. Østerud B, Kasper KC, Lavine KK, Prodanos C, Rapaport SI.
   Purification and properties of an abnormal blood coagulation
   factor IX (Factor IX$_{BM}$)/kinetics of its inhibition of factor X activation by factor VII and bovine tissue factor.
   Thromb Haemostas 1981; 45: 55-59.

8. Owen WG, Esmon CT. Functional properties of an endothelial
    cell cofactor for thrombin catalyzed activation of protein C.
    J Biol Chem 1981; 256: 5532-5535.
9. Marlar RA, Kleiss AJ, Griffin JH. Human protein C: inactiva-
    tion of factor V and VIII in plasma by the activated mole-
    cule. Ann NY Acad Sci 1981; 370: 303-310.
10. Esmon CT, Esmon NL, Harris KW. Complex formation between
    thrombin and thrombomodulin inhibits both thrombin-catalyzed
    fibrin formation and factor V activation. J Biol Chem 1982;
    257: 7944-7947.
11. Stenflo J. A new vitamin K-dependent protein: purification
    from bovine plasma and preliminary characterization. J Biol
    Chem 1976; 251: 355-363.
12. Di Scipio RG, Davie EW. Characterization of protein S, a
    γ-carboxy-glutamic acid containing protein from bovine and
    human plasma. Biochemistry 1979; 18: 899-904.
13. Prowse CV, Esnouf MP. The isolation of a new warfarin sensi-
    tive protein from bovine plasma. Biochem Soc Trans 1977; 5:
    255-265.
14. Walker FJ. Regulation of activated protein C by protein S.
    The role of phospholipid in factor Va inactivation. J Biol
    Chem 1981; 256: 11128-11131.
15. Bertina RM, Orlando M, Tiedemann-Alderkamp GHJ. Preparation
    of a human factor VII deficient plasma. Thromb Res 1978; 13:
    537-541.
16. Veltkamp JJ, Drion EF, Loeliger EA. Detection of the carrier
    state in hereditary coagulation disorders I. Thromb Diathes
    Haemorrh 1968; 19: 279-303.
17. Bertina RM, Van der Marel-van Nieuwkoop W, Loeliger EA. Spec-
    trophotometric assays of prothrombin in plasma of patients
    using oral anticoagulants. Thromb Haemostas 1979; 42:
    1296-1305.
18. Bertina RM, Loeliger EA. The potential use of chromogenic
    assays in the routine monitoring of oral anticoagulant thera-
    py. In: Lijnen HP, Collen D, Vertraete M (eds.), Synthetic
    substrates in clinical blood coagulation. Martinus Nijhoff
    Publishers, The Hague-Boston-London, 1980: pp. 13-23.
19. Bertina RM, Broekmans AW, Krommenhoek-van Es T, Van Wijn-
    gaarden A. The use of a functional and immunologic assay for
    plasma protein C in the study of the heterogeneity of con-
    genital protein C deficiency. Thromb Haemostas, in press.
20. Bertina RM, Westhoek-Kuipers MEJ, Alderkamp GHJ. The inhi-
    bitor of prothrombin conversion in plasma of patients on oral
    anticoagulant treatment. Thromb Haemostas 1981; 45: 237-241.
21. Bertina RM, Broekmans AW, Van der Linden IK, Mertens K. Pro-
    tein C deficiency in a Dutch family with thrombotic disease.
    Thromb Haemostas 1982; 48: 1-5.

DISCUSSION

Chairman: S.M. LEWIS

LOELIGER: I would like to congratulate the Manchester group on the achievement of the BCT/253 as the future WHO Reference Preparation. This preparation will hopefully be accepted by WHO as the Reference Material to which all other thromboplastins will have to be related.

I would like to repeat that also for human brain thromboplastin as widely used by private laboratories, there are three variables in the calibration. First, the inaccuracy of Reference Material calibration. In the case of BCT/253 it is less than 1.5% CV for the slope of the line. Second, the 5% inaccuracy for the calibration of a house standard by a single laboratory. Thirdly, the inaccuracy of batch-to-batch calibration, which is probably around 2% CV. To obtain total inaccuracy of the slope, these three variables have to be combined which results in a coefficient of variation of about 6%. As a clinician I would easily accept such uncertainty in my decision-making in the daily dosage-regulation of my patients.

SAMAMA: I you evaluate all forms, fully carboxylated, partly carboxylated or non-carboxylated in patients receiving coumarin derivatives, you have a lower range than normal. Is this because the PIVKAs have a shorter half-life? By immunological methods we are far lower than the 100% which one could expect if one evaluates all forms of prothrombin. Is there any proof that the PIVKAs have a shorter half-life?

BERTINA: The values reported are the values observed with a Laurell assay. This doesn't mean that in the Laurell assay all the different forms are measured. For instance, we have compared Factor IX results by Laurell assays and radio-immuno assays, and we find substantially more antigen with the radio-immuno assay. It might well be that you are looking at selected populations of the molecules. That makes it difficult to answer your second question because we don't know how to measure the PIVKA so we cannot estimate its half-life.

GRALNICK: How do you know that there is a PIVKA-effect and how do you quantitate it?
I would like to have an idea what the PIVKA effect is. This has been very much discounted in interpreting the prothrombin time but now seems to play an important role in the standardization of the prothrombin time.

Table 1: INR equivalents of survey plasmas (Etalonorme, 1981)

| | adsorbed | | coumadinized | |
	E_3	F_3	E_4	F_4
bioMérieux (rabbit)	2.3 (270)*	3.3 (287)*	3.3 (270)*	2.3 (287)*
Stago (rabbit/simian)	2.3 (202)	3.3 (245)	3.5 (202)	2.5 (245)
Techn. Biol. (rabbit?)	2.3 (78)	3.3 (59)	3.5 (78)	2.5 (59)
Thrombotest (bovine)	1.9 (473)	2.5 (169)	3.2 (434)	2.5 (168)

ISI (RELAC) bioM 2.2; St 2.0; TB 1.7; TT 1.05 (estimated normal value: 38 sec).
INRs were calculated from the survey data using the equation INR=antilog(ISI.log R), where R is the ratio of abnormal plasma PT to local control PT (manual determinations only).

*values in parentheses give the number of participants.

LOELIGER: Table 1 is taken from the Etalonorme results. For artificial plasma (E_3,F_3) not containing PIVKA, the INR
value for bovine thromboplastin - which is very sensitive
to PIVKA - is about 20% lower than the corresponding
values for the other three thromboplastins. For coumadinized plasma (E_4,F_4) containing PIVKA there is virtually no difference in INR between the thromboplastins.

KOEPKE: If we use rabbit thromboplastin, we do not have to worry
about PIVKA?

LOELIGER: If you have very similar rabbit thromboplastins which
are all insensitive or sensitive to the same degree (I do
not know whether they are sensitive or not to one of the
PIVKAs), then you can indeed standardize with the use of
artificially prepared plasma, but only if the INR-equiva-
lent is known.

LEWIS : Is there going to be any difference in approach now that
67/40 is being replaced not by an identical material but
by a distinctly separate form of human brain?

POLLER: I think the PIVKA-effect will be less of a problem because the human brain Quick-test reagent is less sensitive to PIVKA and therefore there must be more uniformity
in results between reagents.

DENSON: I think IRP 67/40 has quite a unique position because it
is a dilution reagent which was made with a very weak
human brain and which is less sensitive than human brain
to PIVKA. It is unique because it has a good correlation
with rabbit brain and a good correlation with human
brain, but if you compare rabbit brain directly with
human brain, in my experience and in that of Prof. Ilsley
Ingram in the ICTH/ICSH trial, there is very poor correlation with rabbit and human. Thus, I am sure that 67/40
is a very good preparation as a primary standard.

If you get a better correlation with rabbit and IRP 67/40, and human (plain) and 67/40, then when you come to calibrate the next rabbit preparation you will have a better line on the international standardization. This is probably why you have a good line with this standardization of rabbit thromboplastin against 67/40. I am saying that Prof. Ingram showed very poor correlation between rabbit and human plain.

TOMENSON: We have done calibrations of RBT/79 against BCT/253, which, on a log scale, are as good as anything you have seen today.

DENSON: All I am saying is that previous correlations have been bad.

LEWIS : Is Dr. Triplett suggesting that proficiency testing can be used as an alternative to a formal standardization methodology?

TRIPLETT: No, what we were suggesting is that the corrected prothrombin time can, with another parameter, be converted to the International Normalized Ratio.

LOELIGER: I would say that the standardization part of the proficiency testing should be used as a check of the normalization procedure.

GEIGER: Quick insisted that unless you have a 12 seconds normal prothrombin time, the thromboplastin was not worth anything. With an increase of the normal prothrombin time you get into completely different curves with different sensitivities and the same is true for dilution of thromboplastins: you can make them "better" and you can make them "worse". Why don't the standards start at 12 seconds?

POLLER: A lot of the trouble with the difference in reagents is that one is just looking at normals and not at the effects on patients. The emphasis here is very much the opposite. Most of the thromboplastins have similar normal ranges and yet are very different in their reaction to patients. Therefore you cannot go by the normal values and you cannot go by normal dilution curves.

LENAHAN: I believe that Dr. Quick obtained his 12 seconds prothrombin time by altering the calcium chloride concentration in the thromboplastin mixture. For each sample, he titrated the calcium chloride concentration. Certainly we do not want that!

DENSON: If you get a rabbit brain with a 15 to 17 seconds normal, it is always more sensitive than one of 12 seconds.

Chapter 14: JOINT ICTH/ICSH PROPOSED POLICY STATEMENT WITH RESPECT TO REPORTING THE PROTHROMBIN TIME IN ORAL ANTICOAGULANT CONTROL

INTRODUCTION

The coagulation defect induced by oral anticoagulation therapy cannot as yet (1983) be unequivocally quantified and reported in biochemical terms. It continues to be assessed by means of the biological assay procedure developed half a century ago by Armand Quick (1) and it can be expressed as time, ratio[1], index[2], or as percentage activity[3]. Quick had introduced rabbit brain extract, which he called thromboplastin, as the procedure's major reactant. Under the influence of Quick's rabbit thromboplastin, the recalcification time of plasma shortened, for a normal individual, to 12 sec. Under the supposition that prothrombin was the limiting factor, Quick gave it the name prothrombin time (PT). For orally anticoagulated patients, Quick recommended, up to the 1960s, to prolong the PT to 25-30 sec (2).

After 1950, many modifications of Quick's original test have been developed and a whole series of thromboplastins of different tissue source (bovine, human, porcine, simian, etc.) were introduced. As a consequence of this development, the optimal target level of anticoagulation in a patient with an artificial heart

- -

[1]ratio: $\dfrac{\text{patient's prothrombin time}}{\text{normal prothrombin time}}$

[2]index: $\dfrac{\text{normal prothrombin time}}{\text{patient's prothrombin time}} \times 100$

[3]activity: dilution of normal plasma in physiological saline or adsorbed plasma, in per cent

valve (a target which in terms of the primary WHO reference thromboplastin is a <u>4-times prolongation of the normal PT</u>), nowadays ranges between 16.5 and 160 when expressed in seconds, between 1.8 and 4 when expressed as ratio[1], between 25 and 55 when expressed as index[2], or between 6 and 28 when expressed as activity[3], the width of the ranges being partially due to technical modifications of the test, but differences in the reactivity of thromboplastin towards the components of the coumarin-induced coagulation defect playing an equally important role.

The only sensible solution to overcome the major present differences in interpretation of the prothrombin time is to standardize (normalize) its reporting by expressing it in terms of a well-defined reference procedure making use of a stable reference thromboplastin. Such a combination is now available. WHO established a primary reference thromboplastin in 1977, consisting of human brain thromboplastin, combined, in terms of which all other thromboplastins/prothrombin times are to be expressed (3). In 1982, on the basis of a Certification Report of Three Reference Materials for Thromboplastin, published by the Community Bureau of Reference of the Commission of the European Communities (4), and based on the results of two international calibration studies (5,6) WHO published the revised Requirements for Thromboplastin and Plasma used to Control Anticoagulant Therapy, providing in addition the protocol to be followed for accurate thromboplastin calibration (7). In 1979, WHO had established two secondary reference materials, one based on bovine thromboplastin and the other on rabbit thromboplastin (8). The rabbit reference thromboplastin was replaced in 1982 (7), and in 1983, WHO is due to consider replacement of the primary reference material human combined, by the proposed second WHO International Reference Thromboplastin, human, plain (6), to be used as the reference material for national health laboratories since long relying on British Comparative Thromboplastin for prothrombin time standardization and as the basic reference material against which all other thromboplastins will be calibrated from 1983 on. WHO will at the same time consider replacement of the secondary reference material, bovine thromboplastin, combined.

The parameter/quantity defining the relationship between the primary reference thromboplastin and another thromboplastin is the slope of the orthogonal regression line when the logarithms of prothrombin times obtained with the primary International Reference Preparation (NIBSC code nr. 67/40) are plotted (y-axis) against the logarithms of prothrombin times obtained with the thromboplastin to be calibrated on the same set of normals' and anticoagulated patients' plasmas. The slope of the primary WHO reference thromboplastin by definition is 1.0. That of the WHO secondary reference material, rabbit thromboplastin, plain, is 1.4. For the second WHO International Reference Thromboplastin, human, plain, a slope of 1.1 is proposed, and for the replacement of the WHO secondary reference material, bovine, combined, the slope will be 1.0.

The WHO reference preparations are available only to national agencies, i.e., national reference laboratories. Therefore, the European Community Bureau of Reference (BCR) has made available for use by manufacturers of commercial thromboplastins and by private laboratories preparing their own so-called home-made thromboplastin, reference materials of different tissue source (bovine, human, and rabbit), certified in terms of the primary W.H.O reference thromboplastin (see APPENDIX). National reference laboratories will calibrate national reference thromboplastins and manufacturers will calibrate a representative batch of their production series, called a House Standard. For these calibrations, fresh patient and fresh normal plasmas are to be used. Batch to batch calibration may then be done according to a simplified procedure using lyophilized plasma, prepared from patients on stable oral anticoagulation (9).

For the vast majority of commercial thromboplastins, prothrombin times as measured in normal individuals and in patients on long-term oral anticoagulation, the WHO model of the relationship with the certified BCR reference materials holds (10). This enables the manufacturer to indicate, for any of the batches he produces, what the prothrombin time ratios found with his thromboplastin mean in terms of International Normalized Ratios (INRs) (11), which are the prothrombin time ratios which would have been found if the primary WHO reference thromboplastin had been used. The equation for translating the ratio obtained with any thromboplastin that follows the WHO model is:

INR = antilog{log(ratio) x slope}.

For thromboplastins not following the WHO model for calibration, INRs will be calculated on the basis of the relationship between prothrombin time ratios obtained with patient plasmas only.

The local laboratory, meticulously following the manufacturer's recommendations on how to perform the PT, and disposing of a normal plasma representing the mean normal value (preferably a lyophilized normal plasma calibrated by the manufacturers against a reference normal (12)), will make use of the manufacturer's table and/or graph to express the locally found ratio into INR. Accurate calibration provided, the INR calculated for the individual patient monitored at an out-patient anticoagulant clinic displays a coefficient of variation in the order of magnitude of 10 per cent, which is far less than the variability (between thromboplastins) of the quantity used at present for the expression of the results of the prothrombin time test, whether it be time, ratio, index, or activity.

PROPOSED POLICY STATEMENT

In conformity with the WHO model it is proposed that manufacturers of thromboplastins should indicate the relationship of their batch(es) to reference preparation(s) by a number of the comparative slope (c)[4] and should provide a Table[5] or Figure[5] indicating the relationship between the conventional terms of expression of results of the PT test and the INRs.

This does not preclude the development or implementation of plasma, synthetic substrates or other methods of prothrombin time

- -

[4]At present referred to by WHO as International Sensitivity Index (ISI).
[5]See Table 1 and Figure 1.

standardization of oral anticoagulant therapy in the future. In calculating in INR it is important to consider the effect(s) of pre-test variables and the type of the instrumentation used in the PT determination.

Table 1: Example of a manufacturer's table for translating a patient's prothrombin time into INR

| patient's prothrombin time: 18 sec |
| normal prothrombin time: 12 sec |

ISI = 2.3

prothrombin time ratio	PT index	percent activity	INR
1.0	100	100	1.0
1.1	91	74	1.2
1.2	83	57	1.5
1.3	77	48	1.8
1.4	71	41	2.2
1.5	67	35	2.5
1.6	62	31	2.9
1.7	59	28	3.4
1.8	56	25	3.9
1.9	53	23	4.4
2.0	50	21	4.9
2.1	48	20	5.5
2.2	45	18.5	6.1
2.3	43	17.4	6.8
2.4	42	16.4	7.5
2.5	40	15.4	8.2
2.6	38	14.6	9.0
2.7	37	13.9	9.8
2.8	36	13.2	10.7
2.9	34	12.6	11.6
3.0	33	12.0	12.5

Users of commercially available thromboplastin preparations are urged to follow the manufacturer s recommendations for use of the slope (c) of the thromboplastin to calculate the INR, and to include this measurement along with their traditional measurement in their report (only on patients receiving oral anticoagulant therapy). This is especially important in the case of any patient who is likely to be referred to another laboratory where a

246

different modification of the prothrombin time test may be used for anticoagulant control. The local laboratory should provide such patients with the INR value as well as with the usual (seconds, percentage activity, or ratio) measurement used in each laboratory of their tested plasma.

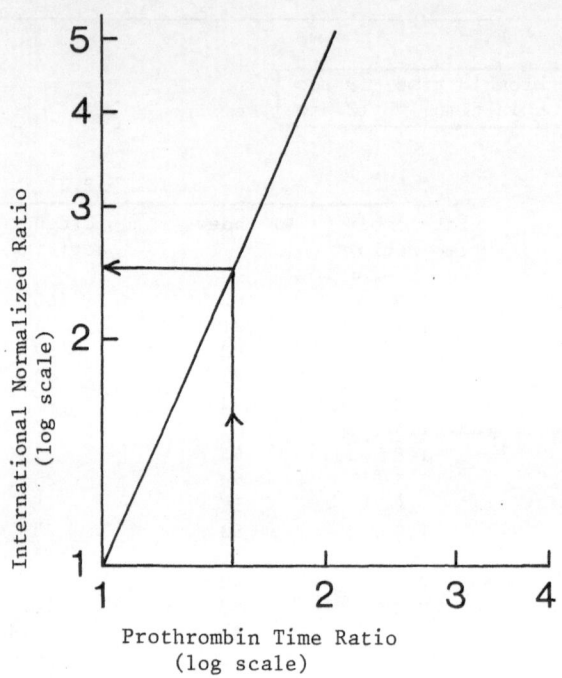

FIGURE 1: Example of a manufacturer's graph for translating a patient's prothrombin time ratio into INR

Investigators are urged to take into consideration INRs when dealing with intensity of oral anticoagulation. Editors and reviewers of scientific papers are urged not to accept the expression of prothrombin times which are given only in traditional terms. Teachers are also urged to adopt the new system when instructing students.

REFERENCES

1. Quick AJ, Leu M. Quantitative determination of prothrombin. J Biol Chem 1937; 119:81.
2. Quick AJ. Clinical interpretation of the one-stage prothrombin time. Circulation 1961; 24:1422.
3. WHO Expert Committee on Biological Standardization. 28th Report. WHO Technical Report Series 610: pp. 14-15 and 45-51. World Health Organization, Geneva 1977.
4. Loeliger EA, Van den Besselaar AMHP, Hermans J, Van der Velde EA. Certification of three reference materials for thromboplastins. BCR information. Bureau Communautaire de Référence, Brussels 1981.
5. Hermans J, Van den Besselaar AMHP, Loeliger EA, Van der Velde EA. A collaborative calibration study of reference materials for thromboplastins. Thromb Haemostas 1983; 50: 712-717.
6. Thomson JM, Stevenson KJ, Tomenson JA. Report on proposed second WHO international reference thromboplastin, human, plain, to replace the WHO international reference preparation, human, combined. Submitted to WHO 1983.
7. WHO Expert Committee on Biological Standardization. 33rd Report. WHO Technical Report Series 687: pp. 25 and 81-105. World Health Organization, Geneva 1983.
8. WHO Expert Committee on Biological Standardization. 30th Report. WHO Technical Report Series 638: p. 23. World Health Organization, Geneva 1979.
9. Van den Besselaar AMHP, Van Halem-Visser LP, Hoekstra-Schuman M, Van der Marel-van Nieuwkoop W, Loeliger EA. Simplified thromboplastin calibration. Further experience of the Dutch Reference Laboratory for Anticoagulant Control. Thromb Haemostas 1980; 43:53.
10. Van den Besselaar AMHP, Van der Velde EA. The manufacturers' calibration study. This volume, chapter 7.
11. Loeliger EA, Lewis SM. Progress in laboratory control of oral anticoagulants. Lancet 1982; 2:318.
12. Deutsches Institut für Normung e.V. DIN 58939, Teil 1: Gerinnungsanalytik Referenzplasma. Begriffe, Anforderungen, Herstellung. Beuth Verlag GmbH, Berlin 1979.

APPENDIX

The WHO reference material is available for national agencies at the Central Laboratory for Blood Transfusion, Plesmanlaan 125, 1066 CX Amsterdam, The Netherlands. Certified BCR reference materials are available through the Bureau Communautaire de Référence, 200 rue de la Loi, B-1049 Brussels, Belgium. The protocol containing all relevant information and important for accurate thromboplastin calibration is available on request from the Dutch Reference Laboratory for Anticoagulant Control, University Hospital, Building 23-A, Rijnsburgerweg 10, 2333 AA Leiden, The Netherlands (see also Annex 1 to Chapter 4 in this Volume).

GENERAL DISCUSSION OF DRAFT POLICY STATEMENT

Chairman: S.M. Lewis

LEWIS : This meeting was intended as an opportunity for a general
discussion and to try to achieve an agreed policy with
regard to the methods for reporting prothrombin times.
There are two main professional bodies who are concerned
with this, namely, ICTH and ICSH.

Both of these organisations will consider very seriously
the comments from today's meeting as well as from their
professional representative groups, and it is hoped that
they will then endorse the statement so that there can be
a joint statement which represents the agreed view of
manufacturers, health agencies, especially BCR, and the
professions. With such a general agreement we will be
approaching our aim of standardization.

In informal discussions with some of the participants at
this conference, it became clear that there is general
agreement on the importance and usefulness of INR. There
was also agreement of how the INR should be calculated.
There was, however, some dissension as to what term to
use to reflect the slope of the relationship between the
working thromboplastin and the reference preparation. The
term "sensitivity index" is based on the use of the international sensitivity index, or ISI, which has already
been adopted by WHO. We are aware that "sensitivity index" might give rise to some problems, because of more
than one possible interpretation of the word "sensitivity". Thus, if one reagent is not as "sensitive" as another, it might be considered to be less satisfactory,
whereas that would be a complete misinterpretation of the

term in the present context. Accordingly, we propose to slightly modify the ICTH/ICSH policy statement, and to replace the term "sensitivity index" by referring to the "slope (c) of relationship of any thromboplastin to the reference preparation".

KOEDAM: In dr. Hermans' paper, the slope is called "b". I wonder why the slope is now denoted as "c". Is there a special meaning behind it?

KIRKWOOD: The reason for that is that in the original calibration model based on the PT ratio plot, the slope is referred to as "b". To discriminate the slope of the log-second plot from the slope of the ratio plot, the former is denoted as "c".

POLLER: Speaking as a non-commercial manufacturer of thrombo-plastin, I do not believe that if I had my material cali-brated in just one centre, I could reliably say what the correct value was. I would have to give the confidence limits of such an estimation.

TOMENSON: I feel that you should have some estimate of the confi-dence intervals of these ISIs. The manufacturer should be under an obligation to give a confidence interval. The only way you are going to do that is by doing it in a few centers.

LEWIS : This document does not indicate how anything is done. This is merely the recommendation for expression. The table and figure in the draft policy statement are an example of how the expression is used.

TOMENSON: I am just saying that you must give an error of pre-cision just like for all statistical estimates; otherwise it is meaningless.

LEWIS : I am willing to include in the text "and an indication of the confidence limits". But in our policy statement we do not have to state how this must be obtained.

DOMBROSE: I don't particularly object to giving the confidence limits, but how would you propose that an end-user would take advantage of the information, and if he is not going to take advantage of the information, what is the purpose of putting it on the label?

TOMENSON: The end-user would not take any notice of the confidence interval, but anybody choosing a reagent, would have a good idea of how reliable the INRs you are going to calculate in the future would actually be. It is no point calculating these INRs unless you have an idea of how much variability there is.

DOMBROSE: That becomes the function of the individual company or manufacturer who assigns the value and is concerned about the accuracy. But if the end-user is not going to use the information, I don't understand why we would want it on the label; not that I object to providing it to anybody who asks for it.

KIRKWOOD: I agree with Dr. Tomenson that everybody ought to be aware of the precision of an estimate, but I don't think there is cause with thromboplastins particularly to introduce something which is not customary with other biological drugs. Certainly it is important that the confidence interval or standard error of the ISI is calculated, and in a particular region this is likely to be subject to control. For example, in Britain the National Institute for Biological Standards and Control (NIBSC) would be interested to know the figure of precision if they were required to endorse a batch of material for marketing. But it is not customary to put a confidence interval on a vial, and it is not general practice in expressing the result of a clinical test to give a confidence interval. Probably it should be, but I am not sure that we need, at this stage, to burden thromboplastins with this extra degree of compexity. As Dr. Dombrose says, it probably wouldn't be used by the end-user of the product.

SAMAMA: If the manufacturers are going to put these INRs in their inserts, who is going to tell the physician how he should interprete the INR? We need some suggestion from the literature or from experience to say that for prophylaxis of venous thrombosis for instance the INR should be so and so. Who is going to do that?

LEWIS : That, I presume, is the job of the profession, i.e. the professional societies and the professional publications. This is of course why ICSH is concerned with it because one of the the major activities of ICSH will be to explain the principles and the clinical significance to the hematologists.

Chapter 15: A MANUFACTURER'S VIEW OF THROMBOPLASTIN
CALIBRATION. I

D.J. BAUGHMAN

As has been stated, thromboplastin calibration has reached a
new level of technical proficiency. During the last few years
there have been several significant improvements in the calibration procedures. Some of these improvements include: the establishment of several different reference materials for calibrating
different thromboplastins, assuming a linear relationship between
logarithm of prothrombin times and analyzing these relationships
with the techniques known as functional analysis. All of these
improvements have contributed to a new level of proficiency.

With these improvements, the prothrombin times with one thromboplastin can be better compared to the prothrombin times from
other thromboplastins. In particular travelers who have been
stabilized at one level of anticoagulation can expect to be main-
tained at that level when being tested in laboratories, using
different thromboplastins. The importance of this benefit can be
better appreciated if the numbers of such travelers should be
documented. More importantly, these improvements will allow therapeutic limits established in one laboratory to be used in other
laboratories using different thromboplastins. With more laboratories knowingly using the same therapeutic limits, the optimal
benefits of oral anticoagulants will be achieved.

One frequently expressed desire is to include in each package
of thromboplastin tables for conversion into normalized ratios.
Although this is desirable, the dissemination of this information
could be published in other ways. In the United States such package contents would be considered a portion of the label and regu-
lated accordingly. Consequently, regulatory agencies could demand
that each manufacturer demonstrate the efficacy of its calibration

procedure. In such instances it becomes the manufacturers' responsibility to prove the validity of the claim with his own reagents. Such a proof could be costly, time consuming and scientifically unnecessary with no guarantee that the final result will be scientifically acceptable. In addition such agencies have defined their own base for calibration. Such definitions may not be consistent with the current thromboplastin calibration procedures being recommended. Until more experience has been gained, manufacturers are not enthusiastic about endorsing recommendations with such potentially expensive and uncertain proposals. Since it is possible to achieve most of the standardization goals by publishing the calibration results in a variety of other forms, I strongly suggest that for the time being one recommend the results be published without specifying how.

In addition to the potential problems associated with labeling, there are certain commercial aspects associated with international calibration or standardization which should be emphasized. For manufacturers to support such recommendations, they invariably ask, what is the cost and what are the benefits? Table I summarizes one view of the commercial advantages and disadvantages associated with standardization. The advantages include:

1. Commercial manufacturers are always glad to have the performance of their reagents improved. Improved reagent performance would be expected because physicians who use calibrated reagents would have fewer patients outside their chosen therapeutic limits. This would be particularly true if one physician had patients monitored by two or more laboratories using different thromboplastins. Thus calibrated reagents might have fewer hemorrhagic and rethrombotic episodes associated with their use to monitor oral anticoagulation.

2. Increased market size is particularly attractive to commercial manufacturers. Presumably the benefits of standardized reagents would be recognized by physicians, who would treat more patients with anticoagulants. In addition, the use of calibrated reagents would result in the demonstration that more patients would benefit from oral anticoagulation therapy. The degree to which these increased usages can be validated the more enthusi-

astically manufacturers will endorse the costs of calibrating their reagents.

3. Finally, all manufacturers will seek a competitive advantage. Such an advantage could be a more precise standardization procedure or the development of a standardized system with unique advantages. This particular advantage applies to individual manufacturers and is mentioned only for completeness.

The disadvantages or reasons manufacturers would not support calibration are cost related and, unfortunately, more easily recognized. They include:

1. The necessity to validate current tests, or to find new tests which will ensure that future lots will remain standardized. It is a single experiment and will include assaying lot to lot variability. The importance of this validation must be stressed for it becomes the basis of ensuring that calibration of reagents will achieve its desired ends. Such a validation cannot be performed by outside laboratories.

2. Initially there may be additional costs each time a new lot is prepared. If the validation experiment indicates that current quality assurance procedures are adequate, this additional cost may be terminated once the original validation has been verified. These increased costs would include any new tests and the acquisition of fresh plasmas from anticoagulated patients. Such plasmas are not readily available at most manufacturing sites.

3. Finally, the most important disadvantage to calibration is the lack of physician interest in calibrated reagents. This lack is so complete that within the United States and within several European countries no laboratory director believes that standardization is useful or worthwhile. This is even true for two laboratories who are currently reporting data in international normalized ratios. What this means is that those who make decisions for commercial manufacturers cannot substantiate any advantage for supporting standardization of reporting prothrombin times. Thus, the advantages become theoretical postulates with no real value, while the costs remain real. Certainly, if standardization is to obtain sufficient support necessary to achieve its goal, significant physician interest must be

generated. Until this interest is generated, standardization will be very difficult to initiate.

To summarize, there continue to be significant advantages in thromboplastin calibration techniques. To expedite acceptance of these procedures it may not be advantageous to recommend that standardized information be explicitly included with each package in the United States.

In addition, physician interest in having calibrated reagents is so low that most manufacturers cannot identify significant commercial advantages for introducing the increased costs of standardization. This lack of physician interest will delay the acceptability of thromboplastin calibration.

Table I: Prothrombin time standardization

ADVANTAGES	DISADVANTAGES
Improved reagent performance	Validation of quality assurance a) lot-to-lot variation b) current procedures
Increased market size	Increased costs a) testing time b) source of control plasmas
Competitive advantage (more precise standardization)	Physician interest

Chapter 16:   A MANUFACTURER'S VIEW OF THROMBOPLASTIN
              CALIBRATION. II

          J.G. LENAHAN

I would like to thank Dr. Gralnick for including industrial
representatives in this discussion. As mentioned, we have for
many years discussed the use of standard thromboplastins, standard reference plasmas or mathematical models as forms of communication for the reporting of prothrombin times.

When considering these methods, I would also like to remind
the audience of the work by Dr. Gralnick on pretest variables and
also to quote from an individual who contributed so much to this
area, and that is Dr. John Miale. Dr. Miale made the statement
that the successful use of anticoagulants in major centers was
due primarily to careful clinical supervision rather than sensitivity of thromboplastins and to improved laboratory technology.

The manufacturers of thromboplastins have primary concerns in
quality control - sensitivity and reproducibility of the reagent.
Does the reagent supply the clinician with reliable information?
As one of the original manufacturers of a tissue thromboplastin
reagent, General Diagnostics responded to a customer need for
education and supplied a suggested therapeutic range in the insert. This range was the range suggested by the American Heart
Association study carried out in the late 40's and early 50's.
The report of which was published in the early 50's with Dr.
Irving Wright as the editor. The insert in the United States no
longer refers to the therapeutic range. Our inserts in Europe
continued the therapeutic range for a longer time, again, because
the customer demands.

We certainly want to cooperate with this committee and with
other international committees to meet the needs of all cus-
tomers, clinicians, users of the reagent and certainly for

better communication and patient care. However, we ask that any recommendations that are made be clinically useful, show equity among manufacturers, recognize the educational demands that may come with these recommendations, show reasonableness with costs, and that various labeling regulations with various countries be considered.

I would like to close with a reminder that a few years ago an international committee recommended that standard units be adopted in hematology. At least in the United States, these standard units have not been used because the clinician does not understand them and feels no need for them. Whatever we do, we must do in a form that can be presented where needed and eliminated in areas where the additional information might cause more confusion.

INDEX OF SUBJECTS